Praise for ON SECOND THOUGHT

"This is the definitive read on mixed feelings: why we have them, how to change them, and when to accept them. Dr. Miller is a trailblazer in psychology—he combines a scientist's expertise with a therapist's empathy, and I have no ambivalence about recommending his book. His wisdom will stay with you long after you've finished the last page."

—Adam Grant, PhD, author of *Think Again*

"Reflecting Dr. Miller's expertise and his passion for understanding the human condition, this book takes a deep dive into human decision making. When our choices are loaded with implications, ambivalence can be stressful or even paralyzing. But we can also learn from it. Dr. Miller explains that ambivalence is a virtue, and invites us to think about it in productive new ways."

—Molly Magill, LICSW, PhD, Brown University
School of Public Health

"I love the way Dr. Miller uses personal stories to show that ambivalence isn't just an abstract phenomenon; it is essential to decision making. Anyone who reads this remarkable book will quickly begin to apply its content to their own life, from pivotal turning points at different junctures in their past to choices they need to make today."

—Don Kuhl, MS, Founder,
The Change Companies

ON SECOND THOUGHT

Also Available

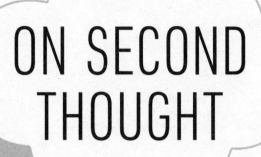

ON SECOND THOUGHT

HOW AMBIVALENCE SHAPES YOUR LIFE

William R. Miller, PhD

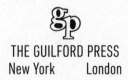

THE GUILFORD PRESS
New York   London

Copyright © 2022 The Guilford Press
A Division of Guilford Publications, Inc.
370 Seventh Avenue, Suite 1200, New York, NY 10001
www.guilford.com

The information in this volume is not intended as a substitute for
consultation with health care professionals. Each individual's health
concerns should be evaluated by a qualified professional.

Printed in the United States of America

Last digit is print number: 9   8   7   6   5   4   3   2   1

Library of Congress Cataloging-in-Publication Data is available
from the publisher.

ISBN 978-1-4625-4750-0 (paperback) — ISBN 978-1-4625-4808-8
(hardcover)

In loving memory of Professor Hal Arkowitz

Contents

Contents

PART III
Working Through Ambivalence

Preface

Ambivalence is our constant companion. It can be thought of as a nuisance and something best avoided, yet it is virtually unavoidable when countless choices are part of daily life. The more I have studied and pondered it, the more I have come to think of ambivalence as a virtue.

I realize in retrospect that I have been studying this topic for more than half a century, although I didn't always name it as such. In the 1960s I was interested in the psychology of humor, which often tweaks ambivalence. My master's thesis with Hal Arkowitz focused on social anxiety, a common experience of both desiring and dreading social interaction. Then in 1973 I began researching and treating addictions, concentrating first on alcohol use, and then expanding to drug use disorders in general as well as behavioral addictions such as gambling. I first described motivational interviewing (MI) in 1983 as an empathic way of having conversations about change. My coauthor Steve Rollnick helped me frame ambivalence as the central issue being addressed with MI—both wanting and not wanting something at the same time. It turns out that ambivalence is a key not only in treating addictions, but in many other professional spheres. MI quickly spread into health care and the management of chronic medical problems like diabetes and hypertension. Soon it began being applied in psychotherapy, social work, corrections, dentistry, education, sports, and leadership. It has spread around the world, now being taught and practiced in at least 60 languages on six continents and studied in over 1,600 clinical trials.

I have wondered what accounts for this surprising level of interest in MI. It seems we touched on something fundamental about human nature. Ambivalence is indeed a universal human experience. As complex creatures in an information society, we experience multiple and often conflicting motivations. I have read the fascinating research literature on ambivalence, and it turns out we do know quite a lot about it. Ambivalence is with us always, and the large and small choices we make in the face of it shape who we are as individuals and as a people. It is folk wisdom:

Mind your thoughts, they become your words.
Mind your words, they become your actions.
Mind your actions, they become your habits.
Mind your habits, they become your character.
Mind your character, it becomes your destiny.

Ambivalence is not something to be avoided, nor can it be. It is the human condition that daily experience involves conflicting motives, individually and collectively, and that what you choose to do matters. It does not always need to be resolved; sometimes you decide to live with and balance the seeming opposites. Yet some of life's most important choices are made in the midst of ambivalence, the hearth in which character is forged. Being more conscious of your own ambivalence is a path to knowing yourself better and to being more intentional in how you respond to it.

ON SECOND THOUGHT

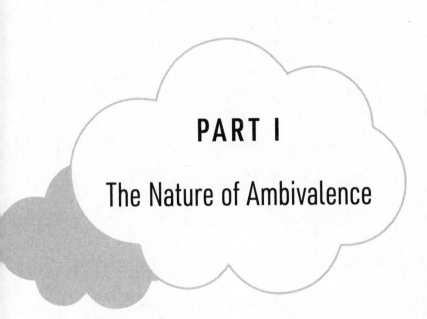

PART I

The Nature of Ambivalence

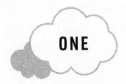

I Want It and I Don't

Tom was the second of six children in a well-to-do, devoutly Christian family. He attended a private school and then a prominent university to become a lawyer, following in his father's footsteps. He married Jane and they had four children before her untimely death six years later, after which Tom quickly remarried, far too soon in his friends' opinion.

He was always interested in government and worked his way up through various supportive roles before gaining office in the legislative branch. He soon ingratiated himself to the nation's chief executive, becoming a trusted friend and advisor. They dined and drank together, enjoying each other's company, though they were quite different men in many ways. The chief professed but rarely practiced his faith, whereas Tom remained deeply religious. Tom was faithful to both of his wives, and was scandalized by his friend's blatant infidelities, though he never said so. In addition to being a gifted attorney, he was widely recognized to be an honest and mild-mannered man, whereas the chief was unapologetically self-centered and vindictive.

Tom became a capable diplomat and then was appointed as the nation's attorney general. The chief's appointment of him was somewhat impulsive, and they had not fully discussed what would be expected of him in this role. It turned out that the chief had assumed Tom would support him in ethically questionable if not downright illegal pursuits. Tom balked. He was torn between loyalty to his friend and country, the duties of his office, and commitment to the precepts of his lifelong faith. When the chief remarried, Tom did not attend the wedding ceremony, and their relationship deteriorated. He maintained loyal silence, never speaking out against his friend, but refusing or resisting actions that he found to be objectionable. The chief kept up relentless pressure and became publicly critical of Tom, who ultimately resigned.

But that was not sufficient punishment. The public denunciation continued, and Tom knew better than to reply in kind. His reputation was ruined, his family suffered financially, and finally he was arrested and imprisoned for disloyalty. Still he did not speak out against his commander in chief. Various charges were brought against him by a corrupt judicial branch, and after three years of incarceration his health began to fail at age 57. The court of Henry VIII persisted with interrogations until at last, based on false testimony, Sir Thomas More was convicted of treason and beheaded on July 6, 1535.

■ ■ ■

Ambivalence is inherent in our human nature, and in a way it defines our humanity. It is our ordinary daily experience to have inconsistent thoughts and feelings. Like music, life might be simpler without dissonance, but it would be far less interesting. An engaging part of drama is the tension that arises between or within characters. Will Hamlet decide to be or not to be, to act or not act? Will the ghosts soften Ebenezer Scrooge's hard heart? The drama of ambivalence is a normal part of life around us. Will a friend stay in or leave what appears to be a disastrous relationship? Having been offered a better job, will a coworker or loved one move to another city?

The concept, if not the experience of ambivalence, is surprisingly modern. Technically, no one was ambivalent before 1910, when the Swiss psychiatrist Eugen Bleuler coined the term that was subsequently popularized by Sigmund Freud. Prior to World War II, inner conflicts in fiction were often dissociated into separate characters like Robert Louis Stevenson's *Dr. Jekyll and Mr. Hyde* or Edgar Allan Poe's *William Wilson,* as though both aspects could not be simultaneously present within one person.[1] As the concept of ambivalence became popularized, however, literature began to reflect and even focus on characters' inner turmoil from coexisting and conflicting motives.

The coined term *ambivalence* combined the Latin *ambi* (meaning "two" or "both") and the German *valenz* connoting power: two potent motives of similar strength. It is different from *indifference* (not caring, having no interest or opinion), *ignorance* (not knowing), and *ambiguity* (having insufficient information).[2] The ambivalent person both knows and cares and is simultaneously drawn in different directions. Part of you wants one thing, and at the same time another part wants something different. Actually, you can be pulled in more than two different directions: *multivalence.* Modern life can pose a supermarket of choices.

The essence of ambivalence is to experience conflicting motivations simultaneously. It is possible to both want and not want something, to be attracted and repelled at the same time. One part of you says "Go" and another says "Stop." It is possible to have the poignant experience of *bittersweet,* simultaneously holding joy and woe together without having to choose between them. It is the "sweet sorrow" that Juliet feels on parting from Romeo, anticipating

5

the future. Another bittersweet experience is *nostalgia,* which was once considered to be a medical illness.[3] Often triggered by negative emotions, nostalgia recalls positive experiences and feelings from the past and can give greater meaning to the present.[4] Within the creative tension of such contradictions, you can consciously choose what you will think, feel, or do, focusing more on the positive or the negative.

Ambivalence is a bit like the local cuisine of New Mexico, blending Mexican and indigenous Native American traditions, with particular emphasis on the native chile plant. Its chemical agent capsaicin is a natural irritant for mammals, creating a burning sensation that can vary from mild to intense. The *picante* heat is part of the pleasure of eating this food. In New Mexico, pain is a flavor.

Ambivalence can be a good thing. The double-faced Roman deity Janus, seeing both forward and backward simultaneously, was the god of new beginnings, doorways, and transitions. The tension and release of ambivalent conflict is an abundant source of humor ("I'm so miserable without you, it's almost like you're here").[5] It has been described as a psychological achievement, to recognize and acknowledge one's own ambivalence rather than projecting one side of it onto others.[6] The writer F. Scott Fitzgerald observed that "the test of a first-rate intelligence is the ability to hold two opposed ideas in the mind at the same time, and still retain the ability to function."[7] People who experience greater emotional ambivalence have been found in research to:

- Be better informed[8]
- Read other people's emotions more accurately
- Be more creative, perceiving unusual associations and possibilities[9]

- Offer fair and balanced evaluations
- Make more accurate judgments[10]
- Be open to new information and alternative perspectives
- Experience greater sexual arousal and desire[11]
- Be less inclined to make impulsive decisions and purchases

There can even be a certain nobility in ambivalence, as illustrated in the story of Thomas More that opened this chapter. He held fast to the precepts of his faith while also refusing to denounce his friend and king or to provide an easy justification to be martyred. When faced with contradictions, you can still keep faith with the values that you hold most dear. Human potential for creation or destruction, love or hate, relationship or enmity is forged in the crucible of ambivalence.

Aware of it or not, you probably make a thousand or more small decisions every day and in the process experience at least passing ambivalence. The potential topics are legion: food or drink, a job, a habit, an event, an opportunity, a relationship, or how to spend your time or money. Short-term pleasure or convenience can clash and coexist with longer-term considerations such as personal and environmental health. Health-protective measures like exercise, eating more fruits and vegetables, mammography, and colonoscopy are common topics of ambivalence. Often the choices are small and transient—what to eat, whether to buy this product or that. For people with severe obsessive–compulsive disorder, even small choices can be paralyzing. Sometimes your decision can have long-lasting life-shaping consequences: whether to marry, to have children, to enter the military or a religious order. Temptation, procrastination, addiction, and change are among the many faces of ambivalence.

7

THE INNER COMMITTEE

A common signal of ambivalence is the word *but.*

> I know that it's important, *but . . .*
> I would like to, *but . . .*

But is almost like an eraser, reversing or overshadowing what went before.

> Your performance here has been very good this year, *but . . .*
> Yes, I do love you, *but . . .*

The tension can be among conflicting thoughts, feelings, attitudes, motivations, actions, or deeply held values. It is as if there were an inner committee with members championing different arguments, representing various parts of you. One member speaks, and another responds, "Yes, but. . . . " Still another disagrees outright: "No, you're wrong." The debate can become passionately heated at times. One member is angry, another frightened, and another self-righteous. It can be interesting to identify the voices on your inner committee.[12] Who is at the table? What arguments are being voiced, and what feelings are attached? Which voices are louder or more influential? Does a voice sound like a particular person you have known?

A common topic of ambivalence on committees, whether inner or actual, is whether to take a particular course of action. The ambivalence becomes a question: Should I . . . ? In my own work as a clinical psychologist, the topic was often what (if anything) people would do about their use of alcohol, tobacco, or other drugs. Few people who are caught in the snare of addiction are unaware of risk or harm from their behavior, and the voices on the inner committee can be many:

- But I really *enjoy* it!
- I know it's stupid.
- It isn't really a problem.
- Nobody can tell me what to do!
- I could quit anytime.
- I couldn't get along without it.
- It's part of who I am.

A common inner experience of ambivalence is to listen to the debate for a little while: You think of a reason for making a change, then you think of a yes-but counterargument. After a round or two of this, you stop thinking about it because it's unpleasant, confusing, or upsetting. That cycle can go on for years. Hopes and fears, anger and shame, passion and logic all somersault together like rough gemstones in a rock tumbler, gradually taking the edge off each other.

VALUING

What a wonderful place this is! We have everything that we need to live, and we have each other. The whole garden is full of good things to eat, and we can choose anything that we want whenever we want. Well, almost anything. There is that one tree in the middle of the garden with poisonous fruit that we can't eat. At least that's what we were told—that if we even touch it, we will die. I've heard, though, that it isn't true. We wouldn't really die. In fact, eating the fruit would open our eyes and make us wise. Maybe it would be OK just to touch it. The fruit looks really good. I wonder.

—EVE

What's going on here? Ambivalence is actually a process of *evaluation,* comparing the relative positives and negatives of possible choices. Aware of it or not, such evaluation is constantly going on in the background of your life. It is what guides your decisions and actions.

Evaluation is a complex process. Often value questions are posed in a binary, black-and-white way of thinking:

Do you want it or not?
Are you liberal or conservative?
Which political candidate do you support?
Do you favor or oppose requiring motorcycle riders to wear
    helmets?
Do you like or dislike licorice-flavored ice cream?

Sometimes on surveys there is an indifference option in the middle—"no opinion," "neither," or "undecided"—but ambivalence is neither ignorance nor indifference. How do you answer a binary question like that when you are ambivalent? A middle choice for ambivalent people would be "both," or "I'm of two minds about it," but that option is seldom offered. Rather than an either/or choice, ambivalence is "On the one hand . . . and on the other hand. . . . " An octopus is doomed to multivalence.

You can both like and dislike something at the same time. Understanding ambivalence requires asking both of the following:

How much or *in what ways* do you like or favor?
How much or *in what ways* do you dislike or oppose?[13]

People can simultaneously hold conflicting beliefs or have mixed feelings of love and hate. Mind and heart can conflict: to support but dislike or to disagree and still love. Researchers can ask,

"Considering only the positive things about X, how positive are they? And considering only the negative things about X, how negative are they?" It turns out that these two ratings are surprisingly unrelated: If you know one of them, it doesn't tell you that much about the other.[14]

Ambivalence is complicated! You can love *and* hate, want to go *and* want to stay, feel both joy *and* sadness. The rich inner world of a human being is far more complex than either/or. Social pressures may persuade us to take sides (see Chapter 5), and ambivalence can feel uncomfortable, but it is normal and follows us through all our days.

Although the account of Thomas More that began this chapter occurred five centuries ago, its themes are familiar and timely. Through time and circumstance, several of his important values came into conflict with one another: his career, loyalty to his friend, honesty, duty to his country, his strong religious faith, and ultimately his life itself. Giving top priority to any one of these would force him to sacrifice others. Instead he chose to honor them all, holding them together in balance for as long as he could. Had More simply acceded to the king's wishes, he would probably be a forgotten footnote in history rather than an honored icon of nobility. The story of his life and death is a tale of momentous choice points at which he maintained integrity with both friendship and principles, at great personal cost. The saga of alliance ending in alienation and revenge recurs in modern news and fiction. Henry's insistence on unquestioning loyalty is likewise an enduring theme in tragedy, continuing to pose ambivalent choices in business, politics, and relationships. It is a drama that plays out even now on the stages of private and public life.

The rest of this book assembles some pieces of the puzzle.

What are the consequences (both positive and negative, of course) of being ambivalent? How do people differ in their responses to ambivalence? Can you be ambivalent and not know it? How does ambivalence get resolved, and should it be? What if you feel stuck? How are your conflicting motives influenced by other people? These are just some of the questions along the road ahead.

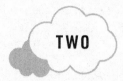

TWO

Four Flavors of Ambivalence

My sweet tooth says I want to, but my wisdom tooth says no.
—Popular song from the U.S. Big Band era

Ambivalence is a normal response to change. Old familiar patterns afford a certain comfort, and yet humans are also hardwired to attend to and be curious or cautious about novelty. Change is constant and inevitable, posing the choice of resisting versus accepting and embracing the new. Your moment-to-moment experience blends stop and go motivations just to get through an ordinary day.

A motive or motivation is literally something that moves you. It increases or decreases your tendency to take a particular action. In that sense, a motive nudges you either toward or away from an object or action. Positive "Go" motivations incline you to seek, approach, explore, consider, be open, or be curious. Negative "No" motives drive you to stop, avoid, flee, resist, oppose, disapprove, or reject.

Motivations come in many different forms. They can be:

- An emotion like anger, fear, happiness, or sadness
- A momentary thought: "I could stop for a drink after work"
- New information
- A physical sensation such as pain, hunger, or fatigue
- A belief: "I should be willing to help someone who asks for my help"
- A deeply held value: "My primary goal in life is to make money"

Needless to say, Go and No motivations can and do co-occur. If you feed urban birds, they will approach you for the food and are simultaneously wary of coming too close. Mixed emotions are not like an acid and base, neutralizing each other.[1] You can experience them both together: love and anger, happiness and sadness, fear and excitement. Such mixed emotions tend to increase with age and experience.[2] Imagine seeing a dear friend for what you both know to be the last time. Accumulated years deepen the layers of felt experience.

Neither do we automatically avoid negative No emotions. People will stand in line and pay good money to be frightened by a roller coaster or horror film. Politicians can actually *appeal* to fear and anger; there is something hypnotically alluring about negativity.[3] Music, films, and memorial services can activate both happiness and sadness. Positive and negative do not automatically cancel each other. You can experience them simultaneously. William Blake observed:

> Man was made for joy & woe
> And when this we rightly know
> Thro the world we safely go.[4]

FOUR FLAVORS OF AMBIVALENCE

Ambivalence occurs when motivations simultaneously propel you in different directions. Go motives urge you toward, while No motives warn you away. Go and No motivations come in various combinations that pose different mental and emotional challenges.

The Candy Store: Go-Go

The happiest form of ambivalence is often a choice between similarly attractive alternatives. It is the candy store problem; the options look good. I vividly remember, as a small-town boy with a coin, going to the local shop that had a long glass-faced case of shelves containing dozens of different penny treats. Which ones to choose? I would wander back and forth perusing the options. Choosing was effortful but pleasant.

Theoretically you could get stuck in a Go-Go choice if the alternatives were exactly equal in attraction. A classic thought experiment in philosophy, known as *Buridan's ass,* has two piles of hay placed at precisely equal distance to the right and left of a famished donkey. Unable to decide which way to turn, the donkey starves to death. The illustration was meant to be humorously implausible, because no one stays hungry at a smorgasbord.

Each day involves choices of how you will spend the time, resources, and talents that you have. With practice and habit, such choices can become more or less automatic: what to eat or how you spend your free time. Each choice excludes other possibilities. A common pattern with addiction is that one option—such as using

15

a drug, gambling, or internet time—begins to dominate and displace all others.

A pleasure in Go-Go ambivalence is anticipation. You can imagine enjoying (and enjoy imagining) either alternative. You can experience a wagonload of Go-Go choices without experiencing too much stress.

> With a strong record from a top graduate school, Laurel had landed a full-time teaching position as an assistant professor, with good prospects for tenure after three more years. [In illustrative examples such as this, names and identifying details have been changed for privacy.] She and her family had settled comfortably in a small college town, and their children were very happy in the public schools, which, if not the best, were good enough. Raj, her husband, had quickly secured a good-paying job in engineering. She was surprised, then, to receive a call from a more prestigious university in a big city, wondering if she would interview for an open assistant professor position there. It was gratifying to be recruited without applying, and her salary would increase. At the same time, she and her husband were content in their current jobs, and she had the advantage of currently being "a big fish in a small pond" where her work requirements would allow her to enjoy family life as well. The options were mutually exclusive, and both were agreeable.

Go-Go conflicts have a win-win feeling about them. Both choices are attractive and agreeable. When one option in a Go-Go conflict is your present situation, the alternative may have a novelty advantage, with the appearance that "the grass is greener on the other side of the fence."

The Trap: No-No

In Greek mythology, ship captains had to steer a course through a narrow sea passage between two dangers. On one side was Charybdis, a hazardous whirlpool; sail too close to that and the whole ship could be lost. On the other side was a rocky outcropping where lived a six-headed, long-necked monster, Scylla, with an appetite for sailors who were snatched from the deck. Scylla and Charybdis became a metaphor for choosing the lesser of two evils. This is a second form of ambivalence: a necessary choice between two disagreeable possibilities. It's said to be like being caught between "a rock and a hard place" or between "the devil and the deep blue sea" and involves choosing the lesser threat.

An unpleasant component of No-No ambivalence is its inescapability, the feeling of being trapped. You seemingly must choose one or the other, and neither looks good. Even not to choose is itself making a decision, allowing the choice to be made by circumstances, someone else, or the passage of time. Here, anticipation in imagination is not a pleasure but a dread. Envisioning either alternative may evoke anxiety, shame, guilt, or despair. Thus, people often put off such choices for as long as possible. When approached by an armed robber who demanded, "Your money or your life," the famously tightfisted comedian Jack Benny hesitated for a moment.

"Look bud, I said your money or your life!" the robber exclaimed impatiently.

"I'm thinking it over!" Benny replied. The alternatives seemed equally appalling.

Ambivalence sometimes causes people to seek professional

consultation. That was the norm in my own clinical work treating people experiencing addictions.

> Matthew didn't really want to be in my office. "The only reason that I'm here," he said, "is that my wife told me if I don't talk to somebody, she's going to leave me and take the kids." The point of contention was Matthew's drinking. He had a good job and had never been in trouble with the law, but spent much of his free time alone in his "man cave." Under pressure from his wife, he began concealing his drinking and hiding his supply, with mixed success. He loved his wife and children, and losing them was unthinkable. He also loved alcohol, and didn't believe he had a problem with it, but now he did. He dreaded the idea of giving up alcohol, like losing his freedom. He also found it unacceptable to lose his family. After several sessions he was clearly leaning toward quitting drinking.
> "So, is that what you want to do?" I asked.
> "No," he replied.
> I was dismayed, but waited silently for a bit.
> "No, it's not what I *want* to do," he said. "It's what I am *going* to do."

And he did. People can choose to do the right thing, even when it's not necessarily what they want to do. It happens all the time.

The Yoyo: Go-No

A third and vexing flavor of ambivalence happens when one part of you says "Go" and another part says "No." What smoker is unaware of the negative aspects and risks of smoking?[5] It is the stuff of country-western lyrics: "How can I miss you when you won't go away?"[6] A peculiarity of this dilemma is that as you Go closer to the object of your passion, the No aspects become more salient; yet as you move away, you begin to long for the positives and minimize the negatives. The farther you back off, the better it looks; the closer you get, the worse it looks. It's like a paddle ball toy, with a rubber ball attached by a long elastic cord. The farther the ball moves away from the paddle, the stronger is the force to draw it back. Yet as soon as it hits the paddle, it begins moving away. This stop-and-go form of ambivalence can keep you bouncing back and forth like a yoyo. Both things are true simultaneously: You want it, and you don't want it. Such emotions can be a roller coaster of ups and downs.

> When they first sought marital counseling, Mario and Maya had been together for 12 years and were childless by choice. Their raucous fights, often followed by mutually rewarding sex, had caused neighbors to complain several times to the apartment building manager, and once to call the police. At their first session, both wanted to complain bitterly about the other, so I met with them separately that day, giving each of them time to air their grievances with which the other was already amply acquainted. She was furious with Mario's jealousy and unwarranted accusations of infidelity and complained of being "taken for granted." He did indeed resent her flirting with other men, particularly when they went dancing, and was uneasy that she had lost a significant amount of weight. Both expressed commitment to, as well as exhausted frustration with, their relationship. In a recent heated argument, Maya had punched Mario in the face, the first time either had been violent toward the other, which prompted them to seek help. She summed up their quandary: "We love each other, and we can't stand being together anymore."[7]

The Pendulum: Go-No-Go-No

Perhaps the most crazy-making ambivalence of all is a circumstance in which you are suspended between two mutually exclusive goals or options, both of which have powerful Go and No features. The same dynamics apply as with a single Go-No object of affection, except that now there are two (or even more). This is the classic "torn between two lovers" scenario. The closer you move to one, the better the other looks. Then as you move toward the other, the flaws become more apparent and the one behind you grows more attractive. Like the inertia of a pendulum, you keep swinging back and forth. As the pendulum moves toward one side of its arc, friction and gravity slow it down until it reverses direction and swings toward the other side.

The adverse effects of pendulum ambivalence depend in part on how long it endures. Sometimes there is a decisional timeline that limits how long the ambivalence can persist, as in the example below. Without a clear deadline, pendulum ambivalence may endure for years or even decades. When the ambivalence involves other people, as with an extramarital affair, the potential harm extends farther still.

Here is an example of a time-limited ambivalence between two options, each of which has strong Go and No features. It is the basic plot of many stories and films, and of countless real-life scenarios as well. The ambivalence begins when an opportunity arises to move to another city, as was the case with Laurel's story earlier in this chapter. Laurel's was mostly a positive Go-Go conflict, but Fran's dilemma adds significant negative aspects with each choice.

The firm for which Fran had worked for 17 years was purchased by a larger company, and reorganization was underway.

Operations in Jackson, Wyoming, were being dramatically downsized, and Fran's department was being relocated to the central office in New York City. There was no position for her if she remained in Jackson, but there was a promotion waiting for her if she moved. She had been to the home office several times and enjoyed the amazing variety of things to do in New York; however, it's a huge, fast-paced city where she knew almost no one, although she would be closer to her parents. She hated the idea of searching for a new job and perhaps starting at a much lower-level position than she already had, as compared to the promotion that she could have. Still, she dearly loved the mountains where she often went to walk or ski and would miss the beauty and relaxed pace of Wyoming. She had many friends and a beloved church community in Jackson, though she was always good at making new friends. She had gone through a bitter divorce two years before, and she could leave behind some of those memories. And then there was Daniel, whom she had met seven months earlier. They were spending several evenings together during the week and on weekends, and she liked him a lot. Were they falling in love? It seemed too early to know, but they hadn't been seeing anyone else and it was starting to feel like a committed relationship. Still, would she give up all the opportunities in New York to stay here with him? He was funny and they had so much in common, but they were still just getting to know each other. Her parents were aging, and it would be easier to help them if she lived closer. Of course, they were doing fine so far, and she was only a few hours away by plane. And yet . . .

Fran's inner dialogue was full of pros and cons of both staying and leaving, stitched together with words like *but, yet, still, however,* and *although.* She had a deadline by which to tell the company whether she would move, so by that date she had to decide, and the ambivalence would be over. Or would it? What if she stayed (or left) and then deeply regretted it?

CONFLICTING MOTIVES

The candy store, the trap, the yoyo, and the pendulum. Most decisions that you make, large or small, involve several different Go or No motivations, some of which may conflict with each other. As I write, I periodically get up from this easy chair for a break. Sometimes the motive is singular, like a trip to the bathroom, although even then there are competing considerations of now or later and whether my writing is flowing or stalled at the moment. Should I run that errand now? Will I get something to eat or drink? This in turn invokes No and Go factors of habit, hunger, health, taste, and interruption time.

Personal and public ambivalence unfolded dramatically during the COVID-19 pandemic, with life-or-death consequences. The novel threat was a virus invisible to the eye, capable of causing severe illness or death, that might be contracted by inhalation or even contact with infected surfaces. More ominously, carriers of the virus could infect others without ever experiencing symptoms themselves. The public health measures to protect each other soon became clear: wear a mask around others, maintain social distancing, wash hands frequently, stay home when possible, get tested when in doubt, and quarantine if exposed. Doing so required major and disagreeable disruption of familiar routines and business as usual. Even simple tasks such as going to a grocery store, church, or restaurant became ambivalent and potentially life-threatening decisions. People responded with a fascinating array of methods for reducing or resolving their ambivalence, to be discussed in Chapter 9. Even when effective vaccines became available, ambivalence remained.

The drama of ambivalence normally emerges in language—whether speaking privately to yourself via the members of your inner committee or talking it over with other people. It plays out as a dialogue of Go and No motivations in talking to yourself or others about change. The motives that get you moving in one direction or another are reflected and expressed in particular kinds of speech, certain words that are readily recognizable because they are how we communicate with each other when requesting, considering, and deciding about change. You already know the meaning of such forms of speech just by virtue of growing up and living in society, where they are part of everyday cooperation. Nevertheless you may not have considered the importantly different kinds of everyday language that are used to communicate and weigh the arms of ambivalence. That is the topic of Chapter 3.

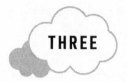

THREE

The Language of Ambivalence

How can you tell when someone is ambivalent? There is abundant research on this topic, but chances are that whether or not you're conscious of it, you already know most of the important clues just from growing up in a social world. It makes sense that over the course of human evolution people would develop ways of reading one another's intentions. Accurately anticipating others' motivation favors success in realms of life as diverse as chess, combat, business, marriage, and sports.

Embedded in the words that people speak or write are many clues about their motivations, including the mixed motives of ambivalence. Nonverbal cues also offer important information and may signal contradictions to what is being said when a person is ambivalent or deceptive.[1] "I promise" can be spoken with complementary nonverbal information (such as hands extended forward, palms up) or with contradictory bodily cues like shrugging of the shoulders. (Look in a mirror and try it!) Aware of it or not, people who are experiencing ambivalence literally *lean* more, swaying a bit from side to side.[2] Chances are you already know how to read some such cues: averted eye contact, silent pauses, or a sigh.

Before getting into specific kinds of language that reflect motivation, it is useful to say a bit about change, which is often the topic of ambivalence. More than an event, change is a process that happens over time. When considering a possible action or change, people ordinarily pass through five predictable stages.[3] This applies to all kinds of change, but for a clear illustration, think about smokers. In the first *precontemplation* stage, smokers see no reason to quit and are not even considering it. Perhaps they haven't thought much about it. As some concerns and negative consequences begin to emerge, they enter the *contemplation* stage. Now they can see both pros and cons of smoking—in other words, they become ambivalent, which is actually a step toward change.[4] Next, if the cons begin to outweigh the pros, the balance starts to tip and they enter the *preparation* stage, considering what they might do and how to do it. If they find an acceptable path forward, they can move into *action*, intending and trying to quit, as most smokers have. Then the challenge is *maintaining* the change. Becoming a nonsmoker involves more than just quitting. It requires some adjustments in lifestyle and identity.

Most human changes are not a matter of "one and done." Smokers normally go through this sequence of stages several times before quitting for good. The initial process of maintaining a change despite ambivalence can be a yoyo between indulgence and resistance. The work is often more effortful in the beginning, and self-control fatigue can set in.[5] Two steps forward and one step back is normal, and over time a change becomes easier.

Ambivalence is richly reflected in what we say when talking to ourselves or others. At least when being honest, the words reflect underlying and often conflicting motivations. Based on research into the language of change,[6] there are at least seven kinds of self-motivational talk that can be used to discern others' intentions, as well as our own. As we shall see, paying attention to these forms of speech can also help clarify some of the riddles of ambivalence.

Why call it *self*-motivational language?[7] Because it not only reflects, but also helps to create and strengthen your motivations. You learn about what motivates you in the same way that other people do: by listening to you talk.[8] In the silent self-talk of thinking or writing, and even more so in speaking aloud, you hear, create, and reinforce what you think. You can literally talk yourself into (or out of) opinion and action.

As with the stages of change described above, there is also a sequence in self-motivational language. At first there is *preparatory* language that you use to talk through ambivalence, sorting out the pros and cons of possibilities. It is the self-motivational language of deliberation—trying on and preparing for possible action or change. Later comes *mobilizing* language that literally gets you moving. I will offer four examples of preparatory talk and three types of mobilizing language. Notice that all seven kinds of self-motivational language can be used in arguing for any side of ambivalence (or multivalence).

PREPARATORY TALK

At least four kinds of self-motivational language can occur as you work through ambivalence. These are things that you might say in talking to yourself or with others. The words reflect different voices from your inner committee as they search for resolution. You will have an opportunity later on in Chapter 12 to try these out for yourself if you wish.

Desire Language

Every language on the face of the earth has a way of saying "I want." Babies learn it early. Speech like this expresses a *desire* for something, with words like *wish, like,* and *want.* Here are some desire statements that you might hear from Fran, whose ambivalent pendulum dilemma was described in the example at the end of Chapter 2. The desire words are shown in *italics.*

> I believe I would *enjoy* living in New York,
> but I *wish* I could stay here in Jackson without leaving the
> company.
> I *love* my friends here and would *hate* to leave them,
> and I really *want* to keep exploring my relationship with
> Daniel,
> but I would *like* to live closer to my parents, too.

Notice that switching of sides in the argument is marked by the word *but,* as if a different member of the inner committee were speaking. Fran wants mutually exclusive things. If she could have it both ways, to "have her cake and eat it, too," she would. Desire pulls her in both directions.

Ability Language

Self-motivational *ability* language says what you believe you are capable of doing, what is possible for you. Some key words to listen for here are *can, could, able,* and *possible.* In Fran's voice:

In New York, I *can* make a whole new start in life,
and I know I would be *able* to make new friends wherever I
am.
Still, I think that Daniel and I *could* be life partners,
and I'm *confident* that I'd find a good job quickly here in
Jackson, given my experience.
I guess it's *possible* for me to be happy in either place.

In addition to the key words, there can be modifiers that convey increased or decreased confidence:

Less confident: I *might* be able to
I *probably* could

More confident: It's *definitely* possible for me
I am *very* sure I can

Reason Language

Reason language has an "if . . . then" factual quality. Fran's story is full of reasons for staying as well as for moving. In essence, reason statements are logical arguments to take a particular action, or not. When committees discuss or debate, members voice reasons for and against a choice before voting on it. Here are some *reasons* from Fran's inner committee:

If I do go, I would be closer to my parents as they get older,
and there are so many interesting things to do in New York,
but it's so beautiful here in Wyoming, and being close to
nature is important to me,
and if I leave, it could be hard for Daniel and me to keep
exploring our relationship.

The word *and* tends to string together reasons on the same side of ambivalence, whereas *but* signals a switch to the other side.

Need Language

A fourth kind of preparatory talk is *need* language. This form of speech has a quality of urgency without giving a specific reason. These statements may contain the word *need* or have other imperative words such as *must, have to,* or *can't.*

> I just *can't* afford to pass up a promotion like this,
> and I really *must* consider my career in all this,
> but I also *have to* think about Daniel in this decision,
> and I definitely *need* to have more than just work in my life.

Need talk emphasizes something that is an important, perhaps even an overriding, factor. "I need" feels stronger than "I want." "I need to be close to the mountains" signals that this is a very important and persuasive consideration.

Mixed Motives

These four kinds of self-motivational language—desire, ability, reasons, and need—often get mixed together. The same kind of talk can occur within a sentence, arguing both for and against a change. Here are two conflicting desire statements from Fran:

> I *love* it here in Wyoming, but I'd also *enjoy* New York.

Two different types of self-talk, like ability and desire, can occur in the same sentence on opposite sides of one's inner debate:

> I *could* leave the mountains, but I don't *want* to.

You can even stack up three or four different motivations in the same sentence or paragraph.

> I don't *want* to leave Daniel (desire), but I *have* to think about my career (need). I *could* find another job here (ability), but I'd be passing up a really good opportunity (reason).

That's the kind of back-and-forth discussion that goes on when wrestling with ambivalence. Some people prefer to do most or all of the work internally by talking to themselves, and some prefer (need?) to talk it over aloud with other people, yet the forms of language are the same.

There are some subtle processes at work when talking about ambivalence. You can literally talk yourself *into* or *out of* a particular choice. Salespeople know this and may ask questions that help you talk yourself into a purchase as you hear yourself speak. There is also a recency effect of the order in which your inner committee members speak. Consider the difference between these two possible statements from Fran:

> I could find another job here, but I'd be passing up a good opportunity.
> I'd be passing up a good opportunity, but I could find another job here.

See how they feel different? As mentioned in Chapter 1, the word *but* is rather like an eraser. It subtly devalues what went before and emphasizes what follows. Substituting the word *and* decreases this recency effect somewhat, although the latter half of the statement still seems to carry a bit more weight:

I could find another job here, *and* I'd be passing up a good
    opportunity.

I'd be passing up a good opportunity, *and* I could find
    another job here.

There is such rich information contained in speech, and this is
just considering the words themselves. Tone of voice, pauses, facial
expressions, and gestures further enrich (and sometimes belie) what
is being said.

MOBILIZING TALK

As time and talk flow by, the balance of ambivalence may begin to
tip toward one side, and certain members of the inner committee
seem to have more persuasive arguments. As this occurs, there can
be a shift in language, and some different forms of speech begin to
appear. For example, Fran might say:

I'm *willing to* stay in Jackson . . . [or]
I'm *going to* accept the job in New York . . . [or]
I sent my résumé to four places in town.

These represent types of *mobilizing* talk, moving closer to resolution one way or the other.

Suppose you ask a friend to do something for you. When you
make such a request, you naturally listen carefully to what the person says in response. Why would you do that? Because the words
that your friend uses contain clues about how likely it is to happen.
Suppose your friend says:

> I'd *like* to (desire) . . .
> I *could* (ability) . . .
> It *would help* you (reason) . . . [or even]
> It's *important* to you (need) . . .

None of these indicate that it will happen. They all signal that your friend is considering it but hasn't quite decided. What you hope to hear is mobilizing talk: activation, commitment, or taking steps.

Activation Language

In the preparation stage mentioned above, you begin to hear language that signals a willingness or inclination to act. There is a rich array of ways for your friend to say that he or she is inclined to do what you have asked. They don't quite constitute a promise or commitment, yet activation talk is more promising than "I could" or "I'd like to." Here are some examples:

> I'm willing to . . .
> I plan to . . .
> I am inclined to . . .
> I'm ready to . . .
> I'll consider it . . .

A statement like this will not suffice as a contract or at the marriage altar. Nevertheless, when talking to yourself or others, activation language indicates a positive disposition, a tipping of the ambivalence balance. Fran might say:

> I'm *willing* to stay in Jackson.
> I am *considering* going to New York.
> I am *inclined* to stay in Jackson.
> I am *ready* to accept the promotion.

Responses like these would not suffice when taking a marriage vow: "Do you promise to be faithful to your partner for better or worse, richer or poorer, in sickness and in health, till death do you part?" Somehow "I am considering it" or "I'm inclined to" won't quite do it. What is required is a clearer and stronger kind of commitment, a "Yes."

Commitment Language

There is a variety of language that signals a promise, decision, or commitment rather than ambivalence: I will, I do, I am going to, I promise, I swear, I guarantee, I give you my word. It is the language of agreements and contracts. If Fran made up her mind, she might say "I *will* be going to New York" or "I *promise* to stay with you in Jackson." Sometimes commitment language specifies a time as well: "I will let you know by tomorrow morning." Commitment language implies that it's going to happen.

Taking Steps

Something else that happens as the seesaw of ambivalence tips toward action is that a person begins taking steps, doing even small things that indicate intention. Someone struggling with depression fills a prescription or schedules an appointment with a therapist. A woman who wants to exercise buys a pair of running shoes. A man intending to quit drinking disposes of all the alcohol in the house. This discovery emerged while we were studying clients' motivational language during psychotherapy.[9] Even before making a firm commitment, people may return for a session and describe things they have done that are steps toward positive change.

TALK THROUGH THE STAGES OF CHANGE

Returning to the stages of change described earlier, language provides clues about where someone is in the process. In precontemplation, when people have not even considered the change or action, there would be little or no preparatory language—no expressed desire, ability, reasons, or need. It's just not a topic of conversation in the inner committee. If someone else suggests a need for action, people in precontemplation are likely to be surprised, not having perceived any desire, reasons, or need, even if they would be able to do it. Before the changes happened in her company, Fran would have been surprised if someone had suggested that she move to New York. She hadn't even considered it.

Contemplation is where ambivalence emerges. Here you start to hear preparatory talk on both sides, separated by words like *but, yet, although,* and *however.* Can you spot the desire, ability, reason, and need language on both sides?

> I think we need to start a family soon if we want to. I believe I would enjoy raising children, although I guess you never really know what you're getting into. My parents really want grandchildren. We could do it now that we're more settled, and if we didn't get pregnant, there are plenty of children in the world who need a good home. It's such a big commitment, though, emotionally and financially, and our life is pretty good the way it is. Yet if we don't have kids, we might regret it later.

You get the idea. It is the "yes . . . but" ping-pong of ambivalence with persuasive pros and cons. As the balance starts to tip, the preparatory language starts to build up on one side, and some activation language may begin to appear.

I think I really do want us to try and see what happens. It's scary, but I think we're ready. We can do it now, and I don't want to look back in 10 years wishing we had done it. I'm even willing to look into adoption. We could start fixing up the extra room as a nursery if we need it.

This language is still trying out the idea, getting used to it. You can hear the preparation stage. What's next is commitment language and the action stage.

OK, let's try and see what happens. I'll stop using birth control.

Of course, not everyone who tries to get pregnant does so right away. What steps and options might they take to maintain their intention?

This example is intended just to illustrate how the language of ambivalence shifts across time and the stages of change. There would be two people involved in the conversation above, and if they were at different levels of readiness, ambivalence would become more complicated. Interpersonal aspects of ambivalence are discussed in Chapter 5.

Here's another example. While I was completing the writing of this book, I listened to a talk describing how it's possible for a person with type 2 diabetes to reverse the metabolic disease by switching to a plant-based diet, essentially becoming a former diabetic. I was diagnosed 15 years ago and my diabetes has been well controlled ever since, but my expectation had been that this is a chronic illness that will gradually get worse over time. What if it ain't necessarily so? To a researcher, the science sounded pretty solid, so I bought and read a text on the subject.[10] This led to trying some new recipes (I enjoy cooking) and shopping differently for groceries. If you had listened to me talking to friends about what I was doing over a period of weeks, you would have heard a progression of language something like this:

Contemplation
- I heard about how it might be possible to reverse diabetes.
- I'm reading about a different way of eating that can reverse insulin resistance.
- I'm not sure whether I want to make such a big change.

Preparation
- I'm thinking about giving this program a try.
- I'm studying up on how to do what is basically a vegan diet.
- I'm willing to try it and see how I feel.

Action
- I'm trying out a different way of cooking and I'm eating a lot more fruits and vegetables.
- I've been sticking with this for a month now and my fasting glucose is already down 20 points.
- I'm enjoying the subtle flavors in soups and recipes I make.

The point in these examples is that language is a primary means for expressing and even working through ambivalence, whether within or between individuals, and it has predictable shapes that you can recognize when you listen for them. Solving and resolving the puzzle will be the focus for Part III of this book, but first, Part II explores how ambivalence actually works in and shapes our lives.

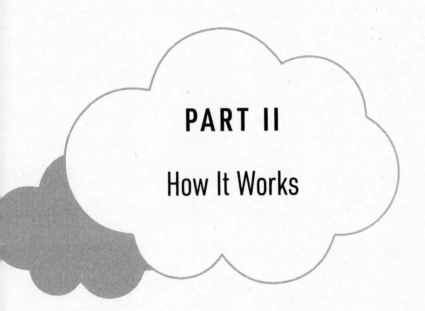

PART II

How It Works

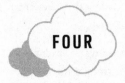

FOUR

Sources of Ambivalence

Professor Milton Rokeach was particularly interested in how values affect people's choices and behavior. In his classic book *The Nature of Human Values*,[1] he reported a series of experiments conducted at Michigan State University in the late 1960s, in which students (97% of whom were White) rank-ordered the importance to themselves of values such as "a comfortable life" and "a world at peace." Of 18 values in the list, two in particular—equality and freedom—caught his attention. The most highly ranked value (#1) was personal freedom, whereas equality was given much lower priority on average (#11). He wondered whether pointing this out could have any effect on students' later behavior.

In three subsequent experiments, students completed the values questionnaire, and then some of them (in classrooms randomly assigned to the experimental condition) received the following feedback based on his prior research:

> Students, on the average, felt that *Freedom* was very important—they ranked it 1; but they felt that *Equality* was considerably less important—they ranked it 11. Apparently, Michigan State students value *Freedom* more highly than they value *Equality*. This suggests that MSU students in general are

much more interested in their own freedom than they are in freedom for other people.[2]

They could compare their own rankings to students' in general and were then shown findings from a recent study indicating that students who had participated in civil rights demonstrations ranked *Equality* much higher (5 of 18) than did those who said they were sympathetic but not participating (11 of 18), or unsympathetic to civil rights (17 of 18). The experimental feedback concluded:

> This raises the question whether those who are *against* civil rights are really saying that they care a great deal about *their own* freedom but are indifferent to other people's freedom. Those who are *for* civil rights are perhaps really saying they not only want freedom for themselves, but for other people too. What do you think?[3]

Rokeach called this feedback a *self-confrontation* experience, because it was done in a classroom setting and only the students themselves knew their own ratings. In essence, the instructions could evoke some yoyo regret in students who did actually rank equality lower than freedom. Those in the control group of all three studies completed the same questionnaires but received no feedback with which to compare their own ratings, nor was any attention drawn to the *freedom* and *equality* items in particular.

Could such a brief one-time self-confrontation make any difference? Students in the studies were asked to complete the same values survey again by mail 3 and 15 months later. Relative to students in the control group, those who had received the feedback assigned significantly higher value to *equality*.

That's not remarkable in itself, but beyond this shift in reported values, would there be any enduring effect on behavior? To test this, a few months after the experiment the same students received a solicitation letter in the mail inviting them to join the National Association for the Advancement of Colored People (NAACP). It was on NAACP letterhead and signed by the organization's president. Students had no reason to connect it with the values experiment in which they had participated three to five months earlier. To join the NAACP, they had to complete an application form, enclose it along with one dollar in a stamped return envelope, and mail it. The rate of joining was more than doubled in the group that had been in the feedback condition (15 versus 7 percent). The only difference between these groups was whether they had been randomly assigned to receive or not receive the values self-confrontation.

In yet another experiment at Michigan State,[4] students participated in the same kind of values study, either receiving or not receiving the brief self-confrontation feedback experience described above. Three months later they were invited by mail to participate in a different study involving a 10-minute conversation with a Black student. Half of the 72 White participants had been in the feedback condition, and half were from the no-feedback condition. As a sensitive measure of interpersonal attraction or "getting along," the researchers measured the amount of eye contact that occurred during the conversation. Compared to the control group, those who had previously been in the self-confrontation condition spent significantly more time in direct eye contact with the Black student.

The behavioral effects of feedback did not stop there. Students in the second of the three studies were the entire entering freshman class in a social science college at Michigan State. Almost two years later, they declared a major in one of five areas of study, one of which was ethnic relations. Of students who had been in the self-confrontation group, 42 percent chose the ethnic relations major, compared to 22 percent in the control condition.

The third of the three experiments had been conducted with the entering freshman class in a natural sciences college. Two years later, about one in four of these students had transferred out of the college to declare a new major. Of these, 55 percent who had been in the self-confrontation condition transferred to a social sciences or education major, as compared with 15 percent who had been in the control condition.

■ ■ ■

It is clear that exposure to information can change attitudes, values, behavior, and life-shaping choices. Although not stated as such, Rokeach was essentially arousing ambivalence by highlighting values inconsistency. The effect was surprisingly far-reaching.

MEMBERS OF THE INNER COMMITTEE

Returning to the metaphor of ambivalence as an inner committee, who are its members? If part of you wants something and another part does not, what are those parts?

Based on his lifetime of research, Milton Rokeach proposed a model of human nature that I find particularly useful in understanding ambivalence and change. He understood personality to be organized at a series of levels that can be imagined as concentric rings, as pictured in the diagram on the facing page.

The most ephemeral, outer circle consists of your immediate experiences like *thoughts, feelings,* and *actions.* Behind these are countless specific *beliefs* that are acquired through and continue to change with experience. Beliefs, in turn, influence and are organized into thousands of broader *attitudes* that are somewhat more stable, but also change over time with shifting experience and

MILTON ROKEACH'S MODEL OF PERSONALITY

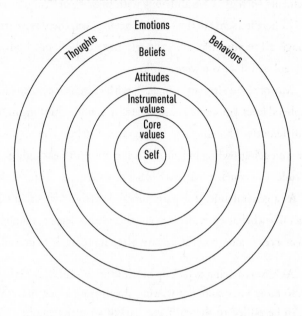

beliefs. Underlying these attitudes, and more central to identity, are your *values,* of which Rokeach recognized two types. First, you have a few dozen of what he called *instrumental values* that are essentially ways of living in the world, organized habits of the mind and heart, such as achieving, collaborating, competing, obeying, and forgiving. These are goals about *doing.* Beneath them are a dozen or so *core values,*[5] the ends or goals that you most treasure and pursue. These are *being* goals: less about what you want to do, more about who you want to be. David Brooks has called these *eulogy virtues.*[6] Ideally, your *doing* goals serve your *being* goals. You will have an opportunity to explore your own core values in Chapter 10. Finally, the deepest or most central circle is your more stable sense of self, who you *are* through the years. This is the observer "I" in statements such as "I am unhappy with myself" or "I understand you."[7] There is a sense of the same "I" having been there as a witness through all of your life, even though every cell of your body has been replaced since you were a child.

Any of these elements can clash with each other. At the most peripheral level, you can do or say one thing, while thinking or feeling differently. Thoughts and feelings can conflict. You might feel your stomach growling but think, "I don't want to eat right now." Attitudes can conflict with each other or with deeper beliefs or values. As a general rule, it is particularly disturbing when an outer aspect like a behavior comes into conflict with a deeper component such as a core value, and the latter is often more likely to prevail.

> As he was driving to pick up his children at the library, it began to rain. They were not waiting out in front when he arrived, so he pulled to the curb and parked with the engine idling. Waiting impatiently, the father began rummaging through his pockets, around the seats, and in the glove compartment, searching for a cigarette. No luck. He knew a shop just around the corner where he could buy cigarettes, so he put the car in gear, stepped on the accelerator, and as he began to pull away from the curb, he looked into the rearview mirror to see his children emerging from the library. His immediate thought was "I think that I can get to the store and back before they get too wet."[8]

The outcome of this true story is that the father, a nicotine-dependent smoker, abruptly quit smoking right then. He had had his last cigarette. What happened was a self-confrontation. His tobacco habit came into conflict with a deeply held value of being a good parent. "My God, I am a man who would leave his children standing in the rain to chase a drug!" Fatherhood won. It doesn't always happen that way, but it's a good example of conflict between different levels of our human nature. Becoming aware of such contradictions can lead to a disconcerting reevaluation of yourself. Attitudes in particular can change in response to such contradictions or when engaging in behavior that clashes with current beliefs.

AMBIVALENCE AMPLIFIERS

Various factors can amplify ambivalence and associated distress. An obvious one is that when the conflicting positive and negative components are both strong, ambivalence is intensified. A common example is the conflict between intense immediate pleasure and potentially serious negative consequences. Sex, drugs, and alcohol are familiar sources of distressing ambivalence, as are the need for and vulnerability of close relationships.

Three other amplifiers of ambivalence are discussed here. They are identification, time, and negativity bias.

Identification

It is possible to *identify* with particular beliefs or behaviors. This assigns great importance to what is a more surface element of yourself (see the diagram on page 43). In essence, such identification establishes a direct link between your core self and this peripheral element, potentially bypassing important values along the way and assigning it special significance as who you *are*. It becomes a way of announcing to the world, "This is who I am!"

Identification becomes especially prominent in the developmental process of *differentiation* during adolescence, sorting out who you are and are not. Styles of clothing, speech, possessions, and behavior take on particular importance. These peripheral trappings of identity can feel important in themselves, but their significance lies in saying, "This is me."

This process of identifying with peripherals can and does continue in adulthood, reflected in how you dress, speak, and act; the reference groups with whom you associate; and how you spend your time and money. Bumper stickers are popular examples, plastering vehicles with reasons to like or dislike you.

How is identification relevant to ambivalence? You may become particularly possessive and defensive about peripherals that you associate with your identity, your *self*. For someone to disapprove of or even question one of these is to criticize *you* as a person, which in turn tends to evoke more extreme reactions. You literally *take it personally*. "To insult my dog [or car, clothing, sports team, political party, organization] is to insult *me*." Such identification can override otherwise important values, so that you appear not to be ambivalent when perhaps you should be. For some Americans during the COVID-19 pandemic, refusal to wear a face mask became a statement of personal or political identity, further heightened by a bit of defiant reactance, a perceived unjust infringement of their freedom. Conflicts over the simple act of protective mask wearing took on personal significance, sometimes escalating to threatened or actual violence.

Identification can result in more stable changes in beliefs, attitudes, and behavior, a process often called *conversion*.[9] Organizations understandably invite identification, so that an individual's beliefs about the organization become self-referential or self-defining.[10] In extreme, identification creates unquestioning loyalty even in violation of previously held attitudes and values. Intentional "sensebreaking" tactics can be used to disrupt and change people's sense of self, creating a new "ideal" identity that is consonant with the organization's purposes.[11] Beyond fostering loyalty, such transformation of identity may favor the individual's organizational or even physical survival, as in military training. Progressive role taking and a shift to self-identification as "alcoholic" is an important process in Alcoholics Anonymous.[12]

Time

Deadlines have a way of intensifying ambivalence, which tends to increase as the time when a choice must be made grows closer. Decisions that can be put off into the future may still percolate in the background but are less distressing than imminent choices. Indeed, temporary relief from ambivalence is an alluring attraction of procrastination. "I'll deal with it later."

When pressured to choose, short-term consequences can trump longer-term considerations. A phenomenon known as *delay discounting* involves giving less weight to consequences that are farther in the future, whether positive or negative. The immediate pleasure of inhaling nicotine can overshadow the danger of lung cancer at age 65. With increasing age, the prevention of potential illness and disability looms larger. Delay discounting becomes extreme in the grip of drug addiction, when all that matters is what is immediately available and any ambivalence about the future is of no consequence. When you can't breathe, nothing else matters.

It is worth differentiating among ignorance, indifference, and ambivalence. When a choice is impending, such as an upcoming decision or election, it is a very different experience to know nothing about the issues (ignorance), to not care about the outcome (indifference), or to both know and care, and be conflicted by the pros and cons of the possible choices. Consider the still-controversial topic of human-caused global climate change. Some people are uninformed on the issue, paying little or no attention to it. Others are informed but indifferent, not really caring about the issue one way or the other. Those who are ambivalent both know and care and can use a variety of strategies to reduce their ambivalence (see Chapter 9).

Negativity Bias

"Oh friends, how few people there are who will believe the good things they hear compared to the ones who believe all the bad things they are told."[13] This was written by Teresa of Avila five centuries ago, and it's still true enough. There seems to be something hard-wired in humankind that gives preferential attention to negative information. Just peruse daily media coverage, most of which is bad news, because "that's what people want to know," that's what sells. It makes sense from a survival perspective, that we would be differentially vigilant for whatever is potentially threatening.

It is clear from psychological research that people do give greater weight to negative than to positive information.[14] I know this well, and yet when I receive anonymous evaluation forms from students, I scan the majority of appreciative ones and selectively attend to the inevitable few from people who were, for whatever reason, less happy with their learning. If I were to change my teaching in response to a disgruntled few, it might unsettle what was working well for the many. Still, I read them, and ponder.

There are distinct cognitive channels for processing positive and negative information, rather than a single bipolar good-bad detection system.[15] This is how it is possible to see both good and bad, pros and cons in a single person or situation. Ambivalence is seldom evenly balanced. Either the negative or the positive will predominate, and the more conflicting the information is, the greater the subjective tension.[16]

When people speak about their ambivalence, it is normal for them to voice both positive and negative information, even within the same sentence, and often with a *but* in between. Even when listening to your own voice, negative information usually receives greater attention. You are more likely to be persuaded by what you yourself say than by what others tell you, and even in hearing yourself talk, you are more influenced by the negatives than by the positives that you voice.[17] It is easier to talk yourself out of rather than into a change. The status quo has a certain inertia, and fearful members of the inner committee can tip the vote. The No motives are generally more distressing than Go motives, and often more emotionally charged as well, so the more negativity is involved in ambivalence, the more distressing it is likely to be.

EXTERNAL DEMANDS

Thus far we have considered primarily internal ambivalence from conflicting values, goals, beliefs, and behaviors. Ambivalence can also arise through conflict with external demands from important relationships and roles. Your own preferences may clash with expectations from family, friends, coworkers, or authorities. With years of marriage, I found myself increasingly ambivalent about our going to social gatherings. On my own, I could leave a party whenever I chose to, and having to stay longer I could feel my energy and interest waning, a common experience for an introvert.[18] My wife, on the other hand, thrives on social interaction and is just getting going as I am wearing down. We both dreaded the discussions about when to leave, and a mutually happy solution was to take two cars or arrange other separate transportation. Ambivalence resolved.

Social roles themselves can contain conflicting demands. A probation officer is both a supportive advocate for offenders and an enforcer of court conditions to protect public safety. Physicians have to balance detached medical expertise with an engaged and empathic presence in caring for patients. Teachers similarly balance fostering competence with concern for their students' personal growth and well-being.

Chapter 5 explores in more depth some social influences on ambivalence, which is an experience not just of individuals, but collectively of families, groups, and nations. Ambivalence is an inherent quality in civil society as we struggle together to balance competing needs and interests.

FIVE

Social Influences

Chapter 4 focused primarily on sources of ambivalence arising inside you, but there are also powerful influences from the people and environment around you. This chapter is about social effects on values and ambivalence.

SOCIETY ITSELF IS AMBIVALENT

Conflicting interests are a normal part of living with others. Civil societies wrestle with how to balance individual freedom and collective well-being. Parents seek to combine nurturing and limit setting, steering a course between the twin hazards of being too permissive and too controlling. When parents and society succeed, children learn self-control, balancing appropriate restraint and self-assertion, which is basic training for living with ambivalence.

Public policy issues are usually about competing and conflicting interests. As a society, for example, we are profoundly ambivalent about psychoactive drugs. Some medication commercials seem to imply that no one should have to experience discomfort:

Take something! Depictions of alcohol in media often have a relief theme: "I need a drink!" Should the use of drugs be regarded as an individual choice, a reason for compassionate treatment, or a crime to be punished? The United States has suffered an epidemic of overdose deaths from prescribed and unprescribed opiates. Tobacco and alcohol are even greater preventable causes of death and disability, imposing massive costs on society. The once unquestioned right to smoke anywhere—on airplanes, in restaurants and theaters—gave way to progressive restrictions in the interest of public health.

Hot-button political issues tend to be about competing interests, often construed as rights. When does an unborn child's right to life outweigh a woman's right to autonomy in choices about her own body? What is a fair rate of taxation for individuals and corporations to contribute to the common good? To what extent should pollution from individual (such as auto emissions) and business activities be regulated in the interest of clean air and water or to reduce global warming? Cultures and nations, like individuals, differ in the relative priority given to personal freedom and common welfare and to short-term versus long-term consequences.

NO ONE IS AN ISLAND

Your own values are influenced by the experiences of your friends, loved ones, community, and culture. A common source of personal ambivalence is when your own beliefs or actions differ from those of significant others. This raises the question of who is significant in your world. There are people whose perspectives do not matter to you; you don't care whether your views are different from theirs. Whose values *do* matter to you? This is often called your *reference group,* a collection of people with whom you *identify,* as discussed in Chapter 4 (see the box on this page). Your reference group offers you norms as to what is right and wrong, appropriate or inappropriate, normal or abnormal. You compare your own behavior, appearance, beliefs, and values with those of your reference group, and when they conflict, it can evoke ambivalent feelings. The larger the discrepancy, the greater the discomfort.

There is a powerful human need for belonging. Your reference group contains people with whom you feel like you *belong.* You are similar to them in ways that matter to you. Similarity matters. There are some ways in which you differ from your reference group as well. With friends or family there may be topics that you know to avoid in conversation because of uncomfortable differences. On the whole, though, these relationships are important to you. You belong together.

Who Is in Your Reference Group?

Imagine a meeting room in which are gathered the people who are part of your reference group, and you are standing up in front. These are people you care about, whose opinions matter to you. They represent what you regard as a desirable way to be. You're comfortable around them, and in a way, you like or admire them. You care what they think about you.

Who is present in the room? Who's in the front row? Name them. They may be living or not, but they represent standards with which you compare yourself. Who else is in the room? Who's in the back row?

A reference group can be formed by shared experience and spending significant time together. Basic military training is designed to create a corps of like-minded people committed to a common purpose. In medical school, the immense time demands and conditions of worth can be encapsulating, fueling fears of personal inadequacy and a desire to live up to or exceed expectations. In Alcoholics Anonymous, common experience forges a strong bond, and members find a "home group" where they belong. Political parties and religious congregations can attract similar people, providing a coherent reference group. Each is a kind of bubble, with insiders and outsiders.[1]

Within such a bubble there can be potent pressures for conformity. In a series of classic experiments, social psychologist Solomon Asch demonstrated how pressure for conformity can override even the witness of one's own senses and reason.[2] Individuals will agree with judgments that are obviously wrong (like which of two lines is the longer) if a number of others have already uniformly given the wrong answer. Stability of conformity is enhanced when a reference group becomes isolated from others and avoids any sources of information that conflict with its beliefs.

EVALUATION EMBEDDED IN LANGUAGE

Values involve *evaluation,* what you care about most and least. Chapter 10 will afford an opportunity to better understand your own values and the role that they play in ambivalence. For now, in this chapter on social influence, consider how values get encoded in the language we use when communicating with each other.

Sometimes values are expressed quite clearly in moral labeling of people or objects as good or bad, wonderful or horrible. Our language is rich in morality terms for straightforward veneration or degradation. Evaluation can also be embedded more subtly in the words we use. A good example is the terminology used to describe someone. Linguistic research in social psychology reveals how the language used to describe personality traits contains both a descriptive and an evaluative dimension.[3] The *descriptive* aspect denotes the extent to which someone shows a particular characteristic of behavior. How readily do they part with money, change their mind, or behave aggressively? The *evaluative* dimension reflects the extent to which the speaker regards that characteristic to be positive or negative. Both descriptive and evaluative information are embedded in descriptions of people.

In simple form, this can be illustrated in two-by-two grids, such as those on this page. In the Risk-Taking Behavior grid, for example, the horizontal dimension is descriptive, denoting the

RISK-TAKING BEHAVIOR

	High risk taking	Low risk taking
Positive evaluation	Bold Brave	Cautious Prudent
Negative evaluation	Foolish Reckless	Cowardly Timid

ADHERENCE TO HIGH ETHICAL STANDARDS

	High adherence	Low adherence
Positive evaluation	Trustworthy Conscientious	Flexible Adaptable
Negative evaluation	Rigid Self-righteous	Corrupt Unprincipled

extent to which a person takes risks. The boxes on the left are high risk takers; those on the right are low risk takers. The vertical component is evaluative: in the top row the person is being judged positively; in the bottom row the same behavior is judged negatively. Thus, people who readily take risks might be described as brave or foolish, depending on how the speaker regards risk-taking behavior. Similarly, the second grid describes the extent to which people adhere to high moral or ethical standards. One who does so can be judged positively (conscientious) or negatively (self-righteous) based on the same behavior. People who are unconstrained by high standards can be described as adaptable or unprincipled, depending on whether their behavior is judged positively or negatively.

MAINTAINING PRIOR CONVICTIONS

Once you have committed to an evaluation in the presence of significant others, there is a tendency to maintain and defend that impression, and deviating from it becomes a source of ambivalence. The very same behavior can be labeled positively or negatively, depending on who is doing it. High risk takers might be described as "bold" if you like them or "reckless" if you do not. A possibly negative attribute in someone whom you like (a potential source of ambivalence) can be relabeled in a positive light, thus retaining a favorable impression. This phenomenon has been termed a *halo effect*—the tendency to retain a previously positive impression by reinterpreting inconsistent information and extending the benefit of the doubt. The opposite can operate as well: defending one's prior unfavorable impression by avoiding or dismissing positive information.

A fascinating opportunity arises periodically to study this tendency to hold on to prior convictions. It happens when a person or group makes a firm prediction that a cataclysmic event will occur on a specific date. Based on detailed study of biblical prophecy, a Vermont namesake farmer, William Miller, predicted in 1818 that the end of the world would occur in 1843, just 25 years later. He began preaching and amassed myriad followers known as Adventists or Millerites. When 1844 dawned, he concluded that God was giving people more time to repent, and he moved the date to March 21 and then October 22, 1844, based on revised calculations, both of which obviously passed without event. The Millerite movement nevertheless continued and gave rise to the Seventh-day Adventist Church, which now claims 20 million members worldwide.

A more recent opportunity emerged when psychologists learned of a Chicago housewife who was predicting that just a few months hence, cataclysmic earthquakes would cause the Great Lakes to flood North America from the Arctic Circle to the Gulf of Mexico at dawn on December 21, 1954.[4] A small group of followers believed they would be rescued by flying saucers at midnight that day and whisked away before the great deluge. When midnight passed and no extraterrestrials appeared, did they abandon their beliefs? No. They concluded that their faithfulness had inspired a miracle and saved the earth.

PERSUASION

Another social dynamic regarding ambivalence is *persuasion*—requesting, inviting, encouraging, or even demanding change. The power dynamics of persuasion will be examined in the next section, on authority. For now, let us assume that the two parties—one trying to persuade another—are of similar power or status and that the one being persuaded is free to change or not.

Our instant-information culture offers a steady stream of communications that can either create or resolve ambivalence. Retail advertising is generally an attempt to persuade people to spend resources on particular products rather than others. Political campaigns seek to create positive impressions of a candidate and to foster negative evaluation or at least ambivalence regarding the opponent.

People who are currently ambivalent (for example, the "undecideds" before an election) are generally more persuadable than are those already holding strong attitudes.[5] For an ambivalent person, persuasion involves decreasing ambivalence by tipping the balance: adding more weight to one side of the decisional scales and/or removing weight from the opposite side. So the thing to do when someone is ambivalent is try to persuade them, right?

No, there is a hidden catch here. Consider that, by definition, people who are ambivalent hold both positive and negative evaluations. They can see both pros and cons; they want and don't want or approve and disapprove at the same time. If you try to persuade people who are ambivalent by making arguments for one side of their dilemma (A), the normal human response is "Yes, but . . . "—giving voice to the other side of their own ambivalence (B). Now remember, they were undecided to begin with, weighing both sides. Suppose you persist in arguing for A, thereby evoking multiple counterarguments for B. You do your best to overcome any objections, but they continue countering. They hear you making one argument, and they hear themselves defending the opposite. Whom are they more likely to believe? Blaise Pascal observed that

"People are generally better persuaded by the reasons which they have themselves discovered than by those which have come into the mind of others."[6] You can literally talk *yourself* into or out of change.[7]

One can also try to *create* ambivalence. A common strategy when advertising products is to tweak human anxiety about inadequacy—not being good enough—and then offer an immediate solution to the resulting ambivalent self-dissatisfaction. If the scale is already tipped to the opposite side (unambivalent), the goal of persuasion is to reverse direction by removing weights from that side of the balance while adding mass to the other side, creating doubt.

In a relationship, ambivalence that is actually experienced by both people can be inadvertently divided up between them, with one partner championing each side. Should we move to another city or stay here? Both partners see pros and cons of both choices. As one of them voices reasons to move, the other naturally raises reasons to stay. If this pattern persists, each may become increasingly committed to the position he or she is defending. There is even something vaguely appealing about this dance, in that they can see their own internal ambivalence being acted out, while only having to take responsibility for one side. If one partner then begins to concede, they may actually switch sides. However, turning internal ambivalence into interpersonal conflict is not necessarily good for the relationship.

AUTHORITY

Finally, there is the social dynamic of authority. Clear dominance hierarchies are found in most mammals, along with nonlethal routines for establishing supremacy and resolving power conflicts. Authority is often a source of ambivalence for those living downstream from it. Few people, if any, enjoy being told what to do. There are situations where clear hierarchies are freely accepted, as in military enlistment or a religious vow of obedience, but even there, authority can be resented.

In human interactions, dominance is often expressed and asserted in language. It can be as simple as a tone of voice that communicates ascendancy. In one study, doctors working in an emergency department referred people who were experiencing alcoholism to receive treatment. At the end of a year they were asked in an interview to describe their "experience in dealing with alcoholics."[8] The audio recordings were filtered so that the words could not be understood, but the voice tone was clear, as if hearing through a solid closed door. The degree of rated anger in the doctor's voice strongly predicted whether their patients had followed through with the referral: the more anger, the fewer patients got to treatment. In contrast, it has long been established that patients with substance use disorders do respond positively during medical visits to an empathic conversation about their drinking and are substantially more likely to return for treatment.[9] In another study, surgeons' voice tone was rated during the first and last minutes of routine care visits.[10] Based on voice tone alone, surgeons who had been sued for malpractice were rated as sounding significantly more dominating and less concerned when talking to their patients.

A well-established dominance dynamic is psychological *reactance*—that the normal human response to uninvited advice is either not to comply or to do the opposite, *even if you agree with the advice*.[11] Why would receiving unsolicited advice prompt someone to ignore it or even do the opposite? What's going on here? Power

Social Influences

dynamics are at play in many human interactions, although often below a conscious level. Through thousands of years of social evolution, people have developed sophisticated maneuvers, particularly in language, to establish who's in charge or dominant.[12] Someone who gives you advice, criticism, or even approval is implicitly assuming a one-up position, and feeling one-down tends to be an unpleasant experience. Persuasion and advice are often attempts to *convince* (from the Latin root *vincere*—to defeat, conquer, or overcome). When someone offers you advice about your own behavior, unless (and even if) that person has authority over you, *you* are the one who actually has the power, because you choose whether or not you will follow the advice. You can assert your own freedom and autonomy simply by not complying or—more passively—by doing so only partially, slowly, and grudgingly. Telling people that they can't do something is not only inaccurate but invites the forbidden.

Remember the studies of Milton Rokeach on human values, described at the beginning of Chapter 4? Participants' long-term behavior was apparently influenced in significant ways by a self-confrontation with inconsistency in their own values. I suspect that the effects would have been fewer, or even opposite, if instead of *self*-confrontation, they had been confronted by someone taking a dominant, humiliating role. "How can you say that your own freedom is so important when you don't care about others having equal freedom? Is that fair? Aren't you ashamed? How self-centered!"

Shame can even have a way of backfiring. Mothers Against Drunk Driving (MADD) have long sponsored what are called Victim Impact Panels (VIPs), in which offenders convicted of driving while intoxicated (DWI) are required to attend a presentation by family members whose lives have been devastated by a drunk driver. The experience can be understandably therapeutic for the victims

61

themselves, who hope to persuade offenders not to do it again. But how would it actually work with the offenders? The gold standard method for evaluating effectiveness is a clinical trial in which people are randomly assigned to receive or not receive an intervention. One such experiment was conducted, in which 813 offenders, all of whom attended a DWI education school, were also randomly assigned to attend or not attend a MADD VIP.[13] These panels tend to be a highly emotional experience, and on exit interviews from the VIP, offenders reported feeling ashamed, embarrassed, and convinced not to drink and drive again. Did it work? In subsequent analysis,[14] attending the VIP did not decrease second DWI arrests of first offenders. Those with more than one prior DWI offense, however, were significantly *more* likely to repeat the offense within two years if they had attended the VIP. The VIP intervention also had no significant effect on a measure of ambivalence and intention to change. It is unclear why only repeat offenders would be more likely to reoffend after experiencing the VIP. In any event, the intervention clearly did not have the desired effect.

Thus far we have been considering sources of ambivalence of which you usually are conscious—your own inner experiences and your interactions with significant others. Now we turn, in Chapter 6, to some sources of ambivalence that may lie beyond awareness.

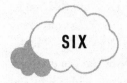

SIX

Out of the Depths

I had not seen the men for seven years. Now back in town on leave, I asked the guys who were still around if we might reconvene the men's support group that had been so important to me during my internship. We had met regularly just to talk to each other about our lives, and now we had a lot of catching up to do.

Foremost on my mind to talk about was an ongoing conundrum. For seven years my wife and I had been discussing whether to have children. The biological clock was ticking, and if we were ever going to have a family, it was time to make up our minds. When my turn came, I told the men about how difficult this struggle was for me and for us both.

"Are you *still* dealing with that issue?" a friend asked. "What is it about having kids that scares you?"

"I guess it isn't really any one thing that I don't like," I replied. "It's just that I don't feel any positive draw to have kids. I don't really like children that much. I just don't have those feelings."

"Bullshit!" It was the man sitting right next to me, at whose home we were meeting. He was a fairly gentle and soft-spoken fellow, and his response startled me. "What was the first thing that you did when you came in here tonight?"

I thought about it. They had two adorable grade-schoolers whom I had gotten to know on previous visits. They were just turning in, and I had gone back to say good night, tell them a story, and tuck them in. "Why did you do that?" he asked. "Anytime I see you at a gathering with adults and children, you're there on the floor with the kids!"

Tears came. Apparently, I had created a cover story that I didn't like children, while my actions were saying something quite different. "But," I insisted, "I still don't really want to have my own. I wonder why that is."

Now, here I need to explain a few things about my own childhood. I have no complaints about it. We were poor, but I never really thought that much about it. There was just so much love there. My mother was an incredibly warm woman, and I adored my grandfather "Pappy," in whose house we lived. I remember a game we played when I was small. I would stand at one end of the hallway, my parents would stand at the other end hugging, and I would run down the hall and snuggle in between them, all warm and cozy. My sister was born when I was five, and we were close. She was eventually diagnosed with childhood diabetes, the complications of which would suddenly end her life at age eight on Easter Sunday. It took me a long time to grieve her loss, and the pain lingers still. I had worked on it in therapy and was fairly sure that losing her did not explain my lack of interest in having children.

I haven't said much thus far about my father. My memory of him was as a sad, depressed, lonely, withdrawn, and distant man. There was no question that he loved us. He worked as a laborer on the railroad to provide for us, and it was hard, cold, brutal work. When he came home at night, he was exhausted. He was just not there really—tired, melancholy, bitter. It was as if the winters had frozen his spirit.

One night my wife and I were sitting on the couch, once again talking about children. I guess I was saying something again about not feeling any desire for children myself, and listening to her longing. All of a sudden, I was just flooded with memories. It came out of the blue, in an instant, just like that. It wasn't like watching an unfolding movie. It was more like a sudden downloading of computer files; it happened that fast. What I got back were vivid memories of how my father had been before my sister died. He had been playful, funny, energetic. He would romp on the floor with us. We wrestled and he told us stories. Before we could afford a television, he had an old shortwave radio that could pull in amazing things from all around the world, and we would cuddle up and listen together.

I couldn't speak. I was sobbing and gasping for breath. It must have been 10 minutes before I could say anything at all. I would try to say a word and break down weeping again. My wife held me and waited until I could explain.

In that moment, I knew what had happened. When I lost my sister, I had also lost my father. It killed him, too. He did live on for another 15 years, but it devastated him emotionally right then, and he was clinically depressed for the rest of his life. What I had been remembering before this was only how he had been after her death, when I was a teenager. What came back to me in a flood was all of my loving memories of him before that terrible day when life changed. How I feel for that man now, going through all those years of deeply buried pain! And I recognized what had happened. Somewhere deep inside I had made a decision that I wanted no part of anything that could do that to a man. It terrified me. It wasn't losing my sister so much as seeing how it destroyed my father, just tore him apart from us and from life.

Part of me healed in that moment. I understood. As an adult, I could separate my father's pain from myself. It's quite amazing how the mind can wall off memories and feelings until we are ready to process them. I had been able to enjoy playing with children on the floor as my parents had, and still deny the feelings. After that I no longer feared being destroyed by the love that I felt for children. The dam broke, tears flowed, and parts of my soul that had been isolated were reunited.

We adopted and raised three children, and now we have grandchildren and great grandchildren to whom I am Pappy. It's astonishing how much pain and anxiety you can feel as a parent, but pain is the other side of love. They come together as a package. We feel pain when we care, because we care. That's just the way we're made.[1]

■ ■ ■

Sigmund Freud's 19th-century insight, that we can be motivated by forces of which we are partly or wholly unaware, is now widely accepted. Clearly, we do not always know why we do what we do. When we lack this knowledge, we naturally make up a story to explain our actions to ourselves and others. Malcolm Gladwell observed that "While people are very willing and very good at volunteering information explaining their actions, those explanations, particularly when it comes to the kinds of spontaneous opinions and decisions that arise out of the unconscious, aren't necessarily correct."[2]

Sometimes—more often than we might like to admit—what we say and do is being influenced by the immediate physical and social environment.[3] That was the genius humor in *Candid Camera* and similar TV programs that place people unaware in situations where the audience can recognize the influence, while the person does not. We explain what we do in terms that are more acceptable to self-esteem. Our self-deception, too, can be a source of humor. In Mark Twain's *Huckleberry Finn,* Huck tells the story of a threatening mob approaching the Sherburn house. As they come into the yard, Mr. Sherburn steps out onto his front porch roof toting a double-barreled shotgun and warns them off. The crowd scatters, and Huck says, "I could a stayed if I wanted to, but I didn't want to."

At other times, the unrealized influence is not outside, but deep inside us. All of us harbor attitudes and biases of which we are, at best, only dimly conscious. More than we know, our decisions and behaviors are influenced by factors of which we are unaware. The term *implicit* has been applied to such motivations that are below awareness. Research on implicit prejudice, for example, shows measurable biases in associations and decision making that do not correspond to self-perception.[4] A bias may be apparent in behavior, but on self-examination the person denies it. This was certainly the case with my own enjoyment of children while disavowing it, a Go-No yoyo type of ambivalence.

Denial can have different meanings. People can be wholly unaware of motivation that is driving their behavior. On conscious self-examination, they simply cannot perceive it. Freud described this as a defense mechanism, to prevent threatening information from coming into consciousness. A motivation may be partially conscious, but when pressed the person disowns it. Then, of course, people can also be quite aware of their motive but publicly deny it. It's called *lying*.

For present purposes, the importance of implicit attitudes is that it is possible to be ambivalent without realizing it.[5] For example, you might be conscious of your negative but not your positive perceptions of a person or issue. It is likewise possible to be cognizant of both positive and negative attitudes that you hold, but dismiss one side as not being your real or true beliefs. Before my flood of memories I didn't *feel* ambivalent about having children, but I was.

VERTICAL AMBIVALENCE

Thus far in this book we have been considering what might be called *horizontal* ambivalence, a conflict between two consciously experienced and conflicting motivations. There is the candy store problem: I want A, but I also want B, and I can't have both. There is the devil/sea conundrum of what feels like a trap: I have to choose between X and Y, and both of them look bad. And then there is the yoyo type: I really want Z, and at the same time I don't really want it.

A similar and yet importantly different experience is *vertical* ambivalence, in which only one motivational pole is conscious, but comes into conflict with an equally or more powerful unconscious motive.[6] These can be particularly puzzling experiences: Why am I doing this? At a conscious level, you may not be aware of feeling ambivalent at all. Yet the unconscious or implicit attitude slips through in behavior. Nonverbal cues can leak information about the less acceptable part of ambivalence.[7] Skillful salespeople can develop a keen ability to sense these cues. "You just have to know when to close," an engaging sales trainer told me on a transcontinental flight. "If you try to close the deal before the customer is ready, you lose the sale. If you keep on selling after the customer has already decided to buy, you can also lose the sale."

As Freud observed, the unconscious can pop up in slips of the tongue. Planning a speaking trip, I called some old and dear friends to ask whether I might be able to stay with them for three nights. I had met them when they were in their late 60s, and now they were in their 80s. As soon as I arrived, I could see that my stay was stressful and inconvenient for them, a disruption in a well-established daily routine. Nevertheless, they had, with considerable effort, made up the guest room and prepared a lovely meal for me on the first evening. Conversation that had flowed easily a decade earlier now felt strained. My offers to help in various ways were politely declined. I wanted to spend time with them but also attend to my work and to other friends in the city. There was tension in the air, but we said nothing about it. On the last morning I hauled my suitcase to the door, a bit tired and relieved, but also grateful for their hospitality. I stepped through the door, turned around, said goodbye, shook my friend's hand, and looking him straight in the eyes said, "Thanks very much for your hostility."

In a social interaction, it is possible for *both* people to be unaware of what is driving their behavior. A good example is the well-established motivational phenomenon of psychological *reactance,* described in Chapter 5. Except at a dull feeling level, someone receiving unsolicited advice (for example, when a dental hygienist advises you to brush and floss regularly) may not be conscious of the power dynamic at work. Likewise, the person giving advice is likely unaware that the usual outcome is the opposite of what he or she intends, and so pushes on with persuasion.[8]

Vertical ambivalence is particularly likely to provoke extreme reactions. People may "protest too much," with polarized overreaction.[9] Fleeing from the implicit motive, they behave in a hyper-opposite way. This can likewise happen when one pole of the ambivalence is public and the opposite is a conscious but private identity, as illustrated by fervently antigay lawmakers who turn out to be gay themselves.

Vertical ambivalence can also yield behavior patterns that are surprisingly persistent with unfortunate outcomes. "Why does this keep happening? Why do I always do this?" I encountered this in my own clinical practice with people who came to talk about repeated disastrous romantic relationships, as if they kept on repeating the same tragic script. Here are two.

Kai was ruggedly handsome, with an affable manner overlaid on sadness. He came to see me as he was considering getting married for the sixth time. Perhaps, he thought, it might be good to talk to someone first. A pattern emerged: He would fall head-over-heels in love with a younger woman who adored him as wise, interesting, handsome, and mysterious. Indeed, he had a fascinating array of life experiences. They would have a passionate honeymoon phase, spending all of their time together. After a while the magic began to fade for him, but she longed to continue spending every possible moment together. As he retreated to get some distance, she grew anxious and more demanding—a demand-withdraw relationship pattern that plays itself out across cultures.[10] Conflict and separation ensued, and then he would meet someone new who adored him. "But I love her, and she loves me!"

While Kai came voluntarily, Julia had some legal encouragement. She was distressed and depressed after her recent breakup from the man with whom she had been living. When he told her that he was leaving, she began throwing glassware at him, including dishes and a coffeepot. In despair after he left, she picked up a glass shard and sliced her arm several times. The apartment manager called the police; two officers appeared at her door and took her to an emergency room. Over time she described to me three romantic relationships with nearly identical histories. She fell in love with men who were not overtly affectionate, but who deep down inside, she could tell, were warm teddy bears. They would get to know each other, become sexually intimate, and one would move in with the other. She wanted to reach the loving man inside, but as she began looking for more affection, he began to draw back. This left her feeling more desperate and demanding, and he would withdraw farther, until finally it ended with a calamitous fight. After several sessions I asked her, on an intuition, to tell me about her father.

"I remember he was gone a lot. He traveled, but whenever he was in town he was usually around at night. My sisters and I were always glad to see him, and he liked to tell us stories sometimes. He wasn't very affectionate—physically, I mean. He didn't hug or kiss us much. We always knew that deep down inside he loved us. He just wasn't the kind of man who showed it. It's like he was a little afraid of us maybe, afraid of getting too close. He wasn't even very affectionate with our mum, at least not as far as we could see."

Suddenly Julia fell silent. It was one of those moments that therapists dream about. All at once it dawned on her that she had been trying to rewrite the story of her father, to have a different past. This time she would finally get him to love her.[11]

I saw several such unfortunate people over the course of my practice. They were passionately, romantically, chemically attracted to exactly the wrong kind of person for them. Sometimes, as with Julia, a clear reason lay in their childhood; sometimes it was elusive. For whatever reason, they kept falling for the same kind of partner, with eerily predictable results. Even insight into the historic reason did not undo their moth-to-flame instinct. My counsel, sometimes taken, was to try dating people to whom they did not feel romantically drawn. They missed the thrill of enthrallment, but realized that the light at the far end of the romantic tunnel was not good news.

Thus far we have been considering the nature of human ambivalence, its flavors and language, its sources and influences. But what does ambivalence do to people? What effects does it have? The story picks up there in Chapter 7.

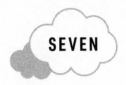

SEVEN

Consequences of Ambivalence

*And being in anguish, he prayed more earnestly, and his sweat was
like drops of blood falling to the ground.*
—Luke 22:44, *New International Version*

To "sweat blood" is a colloquial expression used to describe
extreme distress, often in an effort to complete or resolve something. The allusion is to the verse above from the biblical account of
Jesus in the garden of Gethsemane, as he is torn between accepting
God's will and dreading a tortuous death. There is a rare medical
condition known as hematidrosis[1] in which, under extreme emotional stress, capillaries beneath the skin rupture and bleed into the
sweat glands. Blood thus infuses sweat and even tears. It is a dramatic depiction of the potential anguish of ambivalence.

Yet ambivalence is not necessarily arduous or stressful. I had
initially called this chapter "the *effects* of ambivalence," but *consequences* seems more apt: that which *follows from* ambivalence. As
it turns out, the sequels of ambivalence can be (how appropriate!)
both positive and negative. Some, like emotional reactions, are

ephemeral. The choices that you make in the midst of ambivalence can have more enduring results.

EMOTIONAL REACTIONS

The first emotions that you might associate with ambivalence are negative in tone: frustration, anxiety, and feeling torn.[2] Prolonged exposure to Go-No approach-avoidance ambivalence in particular can yield depression, physical symptoms, and life dissatisfaction. Your distance in time from the need to decide also matters. When the necessity to choose is far off in the future, ambivalence is usually less troubling. Intensity of distress may increase substantially as the time approaches to choose, commit, or take a stance.

In the Go-No (yoyo and pendulum) types, ambivalence can be defined "objectively" by comparing the relative strength of a person's positive and negative motivations. For example, a smoker could rate on 10-point scales:

> "Considering only the *positive* things about smoking, how positive are they?"
> "Considering only the *negative* things about smoking, how negative are they?"

The relative strength of positives and negatives is a numeric measure of ambivalence. With candy store Go-Go ambivalence it would be the relative strength of positive options, and with No-No trap ambivalence it's the relative rating of negatives. If one of these greatly outweighs the other, the person is not so torn as when the two sides are roughly equal in strength. However, the objective size of ambivalence is only weakly related to the amount of subjective distress.[3] In other words, objectively you could have quite mixed views about something, and yet not feel very troubled about it. Ambivalence in itself is not automatically upsetting.

This is not unique to ambivalence. Similar findings have emerged in regard to anxiety. It was once assumed that anxiety is anxiety, no matter how you measure it. There are physiological arousal measures, such as heart rate and skin conductance. There are behavioral measures (how anxious you look and sound to others) and subjective measures—your own rating of how anxious you feel. It turns out that knowing any one of these measures tells you little about the other two. People can report feeling very anxious while looking quite calm. This was common among my graduate students when giving their first public talk at a conference. They usually appeared knowledgeable and confident, yet afterward they would tell me how terrified they had been. It is also possible to be physically aroused and not experience it as anxiety. When I was a new professor about to enter a classroom, I could feel my heart pounding, and if I focused on that it was harder to give a good lecture. There is indeed a fear of fear (or at least arousal) itself. Instead, I told myself that I was "psyched" or "excited" about teaching, and then focused on my students. The physiology of being anxious and being psyched is essentially the same. What you experience physically is different from what you think or feel about it, and how you interpret or label it.

Some classic examples of this are found in the early research of Stanley Schachter and Jerome Singer,[4] studies that would now be difficult to get approved through human research ethical review boards. In a series of complicated experiments, college students were injected with a "vitamin supplement" that in fact was either a placebo or a dose of adrenaline (epinephrine) that stimulates the nervous system in preparation for "fight or flight." Heart rate and blood pressure increase; you breathe faster, sweat, and feel shaky. It's the same thing that happens when you suddenly find yourself in a dangerous situation and have to react quickly. Entire entertainment industries are built around giving people this adrenaline rush. In these experiments, however, the participants had no obvious explanation for why they were feeling this way. The experimenters then created social situations to suggest a potential explanation. The participant waited in a room for 20 minutes with another student who was allegedly also participating in the study but in fact was a confederate working with the experimenters. The confederate behaved in either a silly and euphoric manner or an angry and outraged manner.

Got all that? The question was whether the students would interpret their own physical arousal in light of what the confederate was doing. Compared to those receiving the placebo, participants who had unknowingly been given adrenaline reported feeling whatever emotion (happy or angry) the confederate was expressing. What would happen, though, if some participants were told that the vitamin supplement they had received might have some "side effects" like those described above? Those who were informed in advance about possible side effects already had a plausible explanation for their arousal, and were less affected by their companion's behavior. Bottom line: The emotions that you experience are influenced by how you interpret what is happening inside and around you.

How is this relevant to ambivalence? The amount of your objective ambivalence, the actual balance of pros and cons, does not determine how uncomfortable you feel. The degree of distress that you experience is related in part to how you think and what you do about it. Ambivalence can be, but is not inherently, disturbing. Choosing from a menu of options can be delightful or stressful. Various kinds of ambivalence have been linked to emotional distress (such as anxiety, depression, tension, and shame), to physical symptoms and health problems, relationship difficulties, and diminished life quality and satisfaction.[5] Whether the consequences are positive or negative is influenced in part by how you choose to respond to ambivalence.

FLEXIBILITY

A fairly clear characteristic of ambivalence is that people who see both pros and cons on a topic are generally more open to considering new information.[6] In contrast, people who have already made up their minds, who single-mindedly favor or oppose a topic, are likely to dismiss new information that is inconsistent with their current views. In this context, ambivalence can be akin to keeping an open mind. Those who feel two ways about something do spend more time processing, carefully considering the information at hand, which eventually can lead to clearer intention and motivation for action.[7]

Relatedly, as noted in Chapter 5, people who are ambivalent can be easier to persuade than are those who have already made up their mind.[8] Remember, from Chapter 5, how words used to describe the very same characteristic can be positive or negative in tone? In some contexts this openness to persuasion might be labelled as weakness or indecisiveness, but it can also be understood as flexibility and adaptiveness, a willingness to change one's mind in light of new information.

DECISION TIME

Another consequence of ambivalence is related to flexibility, taking time to consider new information and options. People who are ambivalent take longer to decide and are less likely to act impulsively. When you are ambivalent, preexisting attitudes are less likely to determine your actions.[9] You spend more time considering, and thus decisions and actions tend to be delayed. Stronger ambivalence may produce a kind of "deer in the headlights" paralysis of indecision about what to do. Ambivalence can lead people to put off important medical screening, treatment, and other health protection measures.[10] A fellow graduate student chose ambivalence as his dissertation topic. He never finished.

Leaders vary in their inclination to deliberate (literally: to consider or weigh carefully). Would you prefer to have a leader who is single-minded or ambivalent? Think about it, remembering that ambivalence can mean flexibility, taking time to listen and consider the options. In a way, this is a false dichotomy and depends on the situation. Some roles do require rapid decision making. Police officers, air traffic controllers, and surgeons can be called upon to make split-second choices, where hesitation may have tragic consequences. Training can prepare soldiers and first responders to react automatically. Lives might be either saved or lost by taking a moment to consider options. Wisdom in leadership includes discernment on how long and widely to deliberate before taking action.

VACILLATION

Unresolved ambivalence can result in vacillating back and forth between two mutually exclusive options. This pattern has been called *bistability*,[11] like a light switch that has two fixed positions in which it can rest until it is flipped. Imagine a hollow tube that is closed at each end, in which are sealed a number of marbles. The tube balances on a fulcrum like a seesaw, so that either one end or the other rests on the ground. If the low end is gradually lifted upward, there comes a point when the marbles roll to the opposite end and the tube again comes to rest. Each position is stable until something causes the marbles to roll.

Bistability is a possible product of the pendulum type of ambivalence (Chapter 2) where you are suspended between two poles, each of which has both positive and negative aspects that are important. As an example of bistability, there is a pattern in child development known as *insecure attachment* that can persist into adulthood, compromising the ability to establish and maintain intimate relationships.[12] One pattern that this can take is ambivalent attachment, an anxious and clinging style illustrated in the stories of Kai and Julia in Chapter 6, that can yield on-again/off-again relationships and calamitous breakups. Relationships can alternate between together and apart, each of which contains a yearning for its opposite. Addictive behaviors like gambling or overeating can similarly swing between periods of "being good" and outright indulgence.

DISENGAGEMENT

Ambivalence can also resolve into disengagement: "I'm done with _____." The back-and-forth whiplash and the push and pull emotions just become tiring, and disentanglement is an appealing alternative. "I'm sick and tired of being sick and tired" is a familiar refrain in 12-step programs, one route to abstinence from the insanity of addiction.[13] After a series of dispiriting experiences, someone might say, "I'm done with relationships . . . at least for the time being." Ambivalence can prompt a person to leave a job, a church, or an organization.

Insecure attachment can assume or progress into an avoidant lifestyle that generally shuns close relationships. I have had the privilege of getting to know quite a few people experiencing homelessness. For most, it is a temporary period triggered by an economic or family crisis, and even then, the obstacles to escaping from homelessness are daunting. For me, these are the "there but for fortune" people who remind me that with a few different circumstances of birth, luck, or happenstance, I could be in their shoes. I have met a few who do genuinely prefer an asocial life without the complexities and demands of intimacy. In the 1950s they would have been called hobos, jumping freight trains, traveling from place to place, and avoiding roots. The famous monk and writer Thomas Merton longed in his journal to live alone in a hut as a hermit, apart even from the community of his silent monastery.[14] Some people feel loneliest in a crowd.

CREATIVITY

As will be discussed in more detail in Chapter 9, responses to ambivalence generally move in one of two directions: (1) opening up to new information and possibilities in an effort to resolve ambivalence or (2) closing down to new information to reduce negative emotions.[15] In the former case, the experience of conflicting motives prompts curiosity to consider and reflect on how to cope.

Ambivalent people are more likely to see unusual associations and detect uncommon relationships, both important components of creativity.[16] It is the zany wit of the Yankees' catcher Yogi Berra, who advised "Never answer an anonymous letter" and "Always go to other people's funerals; otherwise they won't come to yours." In contrast, a shutting-down self-protective response to ambivalence tends to close out new information and possibilities, focusing instead on what is already known and familiar. Thus, it is not the mere experience of ambivalence that fosters creativity, but how you respond to it.

It has been said that artists must suffer for their art. Creativity may be fostered by experiencing a certain amount of adversity rather than having a blissful pain-free life. It's not that artists suffer anhedonia—a pervasive lack of experienced pleasure. The key, reflected in great art, seems to be a blend of joy and woe; in other words, ambivalence.

RESILIENCE

Negative emotional reactions to stressful events are to be expected. Anxiety, distress, and depression can accompany significant life changes. More surprising and encouraging are findings on psychological resilience: an ability to cope well with adverse life events, continuing to enjoy health, connection with others, and meaning in life. Positive posttraumatic growth is well documented and is receiving increased research attention.[17]

Remember that an objective definition of ambivalence is the simultaneous presence of positive and negative motivations. It appears that psychological resilience is indeed linked to experiencing a combination of positive and negative thoughts and emotions when coping with stressful events.[18] In other words, the presence of positive in addition to negative emotions seems to help people bounce back from adversity. It may not be ambivalence per se that favors resilience, but simply the presence of offsetting positive thoughts and emotions in tandem with the negative ones.[19] The relationship with resilience may also be due in part to other characteristics that are associated with ambivalence, including flexibility, creativity, and disengagement or detachment from stressful situations and relationships.[20]

MAKING DECISIONS AND CHANGES

Although it is true that ambivalence can delay decision making and change, it can also be a positive step toward taking action. As discussed in Chapter 3, the contemplation stage that is characterized by ambivalence is actually a normal step on the way to change. That ambivalence itself can trigger change is illustrated by the research of Milton Rokeach described in Chapter 4. His students may have seen no inconsistency in their values (precontemplation) until it was pointed out to them (contemplation), creating ambivalence and affecting their subsequent actions even years later.

Some of the most importance consequences of ambivalence are not the immediate effects themselves, but the choices that you make when experiencing it. These are value decisions between competing alternatives. A single decision may have life-changing consequences. There are countless engaging examples in fiction. The story and film *Sophie's Choice* gradually discloses a traumatic decision that Sophie was forced to make, leaving a deep lifelong wound.

In *The Matrix*, the character Neo must decide whether to take the red pill (to see an unpleasant truth) or the blue pill (to remain in blissful ignorance). Real-life decisions can also have lifelong effects: whether to leave home, to serve in the military, or to adopt children. A public revelation as a whistleblower, as a victim of sexual abuse, or of one's own sexual orientation may have far-reaching consequences.

Sometimes it is not one pivotal choice, but a sequence of forks in the road where the path that you choose shapes who you are. An example is how people decide to use accumulated power and resources, decisions that can also have enduring effects for better or worse on themselves and others. Characters in fiction (and in real life as well) make successive choices to share or hold on to power, sometimes sacrificing their families, friendships, values, and their own accomplishments as well. Initially sympathetic characters are gradually transformed in the ironic fashion of Greek tragedy to embrace power, status, or money. Some examples from film are Walter White in *Breaking Bad* and Michael Corleone in *The Godfather*. It parallels the grip of addiction: How much are you willing to give up to continue this single-minded pursuit?

A recurring real-life example that I have witnessed is people, usually men, who have developed a successful organization or treatment method, often building it from the ground up. As retirement approaches, it becomes time to empower the next generation of ideas and leaders. Instead, they cling to power. Once beloved and admired, they bitterly resist turning over leadership and innovations, until tragically the celebration of their departure turns from "Well done" to "Good riddance." Of course, transformation can occur in either direction. *Schindler's List* tells the true story of an initially self-centered businessman who progressively takes risks

83

using his money and influence to free Jewish people in Nazi Germany. Life choice can be redemptive.

In summary, ambivalence is consequential. It can have both positive and negative effects depending on how you think about and respond to the experience. It is in moments of ambivalence that you may make some of the most important choices of your life. There are also some significant personality differences in how people experience ambivalence, welcoming or shunning it. That is the topic of Chapter 8, before we consider the various ways of responding to ambivalence in Chapter 9.

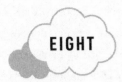

EIGHT

Individual Differences

I was born condemned to be one of those who has to see all sides of a question. When you're damned like that, the questions multiply for you until in the end it's all question and no answer.
—Larry in Eugene O'Neill's *The Iceman Cometh,* Act 1

The term *cognitive dissonance* entered our vocabulary through a psychological theory proposed by Leon Festinger in 1957. Human nature, he thought, naturally abhors inconsistency. For example, if we hold an attitude that is inconsistent with our own behavior, one or the other must change. His studies showed, for instance, that when people speak publicly in support of a position that is different from their own, their attitude shifts toward the view that they advocated. Hearing yourself speak tends to increase your commitment to the person or cause you were defending; you literally talk yourself into it. An exception to this is coercion. If you felt forced to say what you did, then it is less likely you will change your own views.

Yet ambivalence and inconsistency are not necessarily disagreeable. Deciding what to order from a menu of delicious options can be quite pleasant. Some people are untroubled by being consistently inconsistent. Some live comfortably with ambivalence as their normal condition, at least until they must make a decision. This chapter considers personality differences in how people experience and respond to ambivalence. It may be interesting to consider where you are personally on each of these dimensions.

OPENNESS TO EXPERIENCE

A few decades ago, personality research converged on what are called the "big five" important ways in which people differ.[1] One of these five traits is called *openness to experience*. Individuals who score high on this dimension tend to be curious, open-minded, imaginative, and willing to try new things and have new experiences. Those scoring lower on openness prefer to have a set routine and don't like to try new things; they tend to be literal, logical, consistent, and averse to change.

Chapter 7 explored flexibility as a possible consequence of ambivalence. Here the chicken and egg are reversed. People who by nature are high in openness to experience would be much more comfortable with, even enjoy, ambivalence and ambiguity. When you encounter challenging information, are you more likely to be curious or dismissive? If you feel personally torn, are you more inclined to reflect and try to resolve it or just stop thinking about it?

Degree of openness can be more specific. You might be a generally open-minded person, but on a certain topic you hold a strong, persistent, and well-established attitude. On this topic you would be more resistant to persuasion and changing your mind. You would tend to seek and accept only information that is consistent with your attitude.

NEED FOR CLOSURE

Another personality difference has to do with a preference for closure.[2] One pole of this dimension has been called *judging* (not to be confused with judgmental), and the other *perceiving*. People at the judging end of the continuum feel restless when undecided, preferring just to make a choice and move on, even if it might not be the best possible choice. Those at the perceiving end are more at ease with ambivalence, feeling less urgency to resolve it and more concerned about making the wrong decision. I happen to prefer the judging style myself. If I want to buy pants, I tend to go to one store, find a satisfactory pair in my size, maybe try it on, take it home, and I'm happy. ("And your wardrobe looks like it," a perceiving type might observe.) Opposites attract, and my perceiving wife of five decades prefers to consider many possibilities before reaching a decision (which, I have learned, is a wiser style when choosing a home, a vehicle, or a life partner). She goes to multiple stores, brings home a variety of options, and often returns most or all of them the next day. Together these two personal styles can counterbalance each other. One is more decisive and is prone to choosing too quickly or impulsively. The other prefers to examine all the alternatives carefully and may still have difficulty in finally deciding. On a committee or jury that makes important decisions, both perspectives are valuable.

When experiencing ambivalence, the judging (high need for

closure) person tends to feel restless until a choice is made, then is satisfied to move on and is disinclined to look back. The perceiving type is happy with considering all the possibilities and may not be anxious until and after a decision has been made. The ghost of post-decisional regret is more likely to haunt perceiving people; they are more prone to ruminating about negative aspects of the choice that was made and reconsidering positive aspects of the road not taken.

Judging people often need to be encouraged to have patience and continue reflecting. Perceiving people are comforted by having given due consideration, accepting that they made the best choice they could, given what they knew at the time.

REWARD SEEKING AND HARM AVOIDANCE

Then there is vigilance for pleasure or pain. Some folks are much more attuned to the positive possibilities, and when making decisions they are attracted by the potential rewards, gains, and pleasures. The brain has specific reward pathways for anticipating and seeking rewards. When an action stimulates the release of dopamine in the brain, the message is "do that again!" While pleasure seeking is normal in animals and people, it can also go haywire in compulsively pursuing particular rewards, a phenomenon usually called *addiction*.[3]

Likewise, some people feel great urgency to avoid risk or harm, concerned about minimizing their potential pain and loss. When making choices, potential losses loom larger than gains. These people are high in what is called *harm avoidance*. Humans do vary in their sensitivity to potential negative outcomes. Some people are relatively impervious to punishment and don't seem to learn from it. They are low in harm avoidance, tend to be risk takers, and are more likely to continue in self-destructive behavior despite its consequences. People with a combination of high reward seeking and low harm avoidance can be particularly hard on themselves and others, including those who love them.

These two characteristics can influence how you experience and resolve ambivalence. Would you say that you are more concerned with possible rewards or avoiding harm? In the Go-No (yoyo and pendulum) types of ambivalence (Chapter 2), these traits can tip the balance.

DELAY OF GRATIFICATION

In addition, people assign different importance to immediate versus longer-term gains and losses. A famous "marshmallow experiment" at Stanford University asked preschool children to choose between a small immediate treat or refraining from eating it for 15 minutes while waiting alone and then receiving two treats.[4] The characteristic being studied was self-control—the ability to delay gratification. Later in life, as adolescents, the children who had chosen to wait for a second treat were doing better academically in school and were more able to tolerate frustration and stress.[5] Even 30 years later, their childhood ability to delay reward predicted their adult body mass index; they were less likely to be overweight.[6]

There is a related concept in economics called *delay discounting,* already mentioned in Chapter 4.[7] How much does an incentive lose its value when receiving it is delayed? In extreme form, a reward or a treat is meaningless unless it is accessible right now. In the marshmallow experiment, these children would eat the treat right away. Infants are not well prepared to wait for food or relief of discomfort. For an addicted person in the midst of withdrawal, availability of the drug tomorrow can be useless.[8] A small cash payment now may outweigh a larger payment later. Tolerance for delay of reward is a factor in investments, loans, and saving for retirement.

Here is an ambivalence example often used in delay discounting research. If you were given a choice of receiving $100 today or $200 five years from now, which would you choose? Highly logical people might begin computing compound interest rates, but most people choose the immediate payment. How soon would the $200 payment need to arrive before you would choose to wait for it? One year? Six months? One month? Tomorrow?

INTROVERSION VERSUS EXTRAVERSION

When hearing the term *introversion*, a first thought is often shyness, but this widely recognized personality characteristic can have a much broader meaning.[9] Those who lean toward introversion prefer to process information privately. They are more likely to work it all out internally before announcing their decision. Extraverts, on the other hand, tend to work out their decisions by talking them over with other people; they "try things out" by saying them aloud. An introvert can therefore overestimate the finality of what an extravert says. Similarly, an extravert can underestimate the seriousness of what an introvert says.

How is this important in ambivalence? Introverts are more likely to try to resolve it quietly on their own, although they might benefit from talking it over. Extraverts may try out multiple resolutions depending on the person(s) to whom they are talking, but might benefit from some quiet reflection time to get a big picture on their own (see Chapter 11).

NEED FOR CONSISTENCY

So, was Leon Festinger right? Do people in general abhor being inconsistent? The answer seems to be that yes, some do, whereas others do not. Preference for personal consistency is itself a personality disposition.[10] Does it bother you if your actions are inconsistent? Is it important to you that others see you as stable and predictable? Do you like always to do things in the same way? If so, you may score high on a preference for consistency scale.[11] Those who value consistency also tend to be more self-conscious and introverted, prefer to have structure, and are less open to new experience.

Realizing that people differ on preference for consistency (PFC) has helped to make sense of prior inconsistencies in research on consistency![12] If you expect to spend time with someone whom you haven't met, are you likely to rate that unmet person more positively? Yes, you are, *if* you are high in PFC. Are you susceptible to the foot-in-the-door technique: that having agreed to do someone a small favor, you are then more likely to agree to a larger request? Yes, you are, *if* you are high in PFC. Suppose you were *required* to write an essay favoring a social policy change that you did not previously favor. Do you then have a more favorable attitude toward that change? Yes, you do, but only if you are high in PFC. For high-PFC people, being inconsistent creates ambivalence and a pressure to remain consistent. If you're a high-PFC parent of teenagers, beware the foot in the door!

No wonder ambivalence can be challenging! We differ in

openness to new experience, need for closure, reward seeking and harm avoidance, delay of gratification, introversion and extraversion, and need for consistency. With all these needs swirling around inside, the wonder is that some people are so comfortable in embracing ambivalence—a topic to which we will return in Chapter 13. For now, we complete Part II by considering the varied ways in which people *respond* to ambivalence.

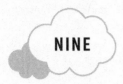

NINE

Responding to Ambivalence

When you come to a fork in the road, take it.
—Yogi Berra

The year was 1219, and Europe's adversaries were the nations of Islam. The Crusades had been a military disaster for 120 years, destroying Middle Eastern cities and countless lives on both sides. Blessed by the Roman church, the armies of the Fifth Crusade had marched off to attack Egypt once again, seeking to recapture the holy lands. In this fearful time, when any talk of negotiation was perceived as weakness, a young Italian priest struggled with his conscience. If he were to speak his mind and heart, he would surely be considered a fool and a traitor, perhaps even excommunicated or imprisoned. If he kept silent, he knew that he could never live with his own conscience. So risking his life, he traveled to the front, to Egypt, to meet both with Muslim leaders and with the Christian marshals of the Crusade, to counsel peace and mutual understanding. He was unsuccessful, as were the Fifth, Sixth, Seventh, and Eighth Crusades over the next 50 years. He failed to stop the war, but he had been true to his conscience and had done his best to promote peace and hope. His name was Francis of Assisi.

■ ■ ■

In addition to human differences in experiencing ambivalence (Chapter 8), we differ in how we respond to it. Although specific responses are many and varied, they tend to fall into two broad categories: shutting down (inaction, avoidance) and taking steps to resolve it (considering, choosing, committing). These parallel more general *flight or fight* responses to stress. It is normal to respond to ambivalence in different ways across times and situations.

SHUTTING DOWN

Sometimes ambivalence can be paralyzing, immobilizing. You don't know what to do, and so rather than making what could be a wrong move, you freeze like a deer in the headlights and do nothing. When you come to the fork in the road, you want to take both paths and you cannot, so you set up camp there. You put off having to decide. It is possible to remain camping at the decision point of ambivalence for a very long time. An intention like "I need to lose some weight and get into shape" can persist for years without resulting in much action. More people join a gym than actually attend one.

Besides inaction, a second kind of closing-down response is to actively avoid or flee from ambivalence and choice. Sighting a fork in the road up ahead, you spin around and go back. There are countless ways to do so. One is to avoid circumstances in which you might be forced to make a choice. For example, a common and often successful early coping strategy when getting free from an addiction is to steer clear of high-risk situations. Faced with a dilemma, you might choose to put it out of your mind or to immerse yourself in work or other distracting activities. Physical relocation such as moving to another job or city is sometimes chosen to escape from an ambivalent impasse. "I just couldn't stay there any longer."

Yet another avoidant strategy is to deny that there is anything to be ambivalent about. There are various ways to do this. One is to remain ignorant in order to avoid unwelcome information. Some people shun medical tests or check-ups because they might receive bad news. Another is indifference: for example, not caring what their blood pressure or blood sugar level is. A third is to discount or disregard evidence. At various times in history individuals and groups have denied what eventually came to be widely accepted science:

- That the Earth is round
- That smoking causes cancer
- That six million Jews were murdered during the Holocaust
- That human activity contributes to global warming
- That the COVID-19 virus is real and dangerous

In essence, this solution is deciding that there is no reason to be ambivalent because it's a myth or hoax. This is maintained by confirmation bias: seeking and selectively attending only to information that is consistent with your belief, while avoiding all evidence to the contrary. If you cannot escape contradictory information, another strategy is to invalidate and dismiss the source itself.

This happens within science, as well, when major paradigm shifts occur that challenge previously established assumptions and approaches.[1] Some historic examples of such paradigm shifts are the astronomy of Copernicus and Galileo, germ theory in medicine, natural selection in biology, and relativity and quantum mechanics in physics. Such scientific revolutions are ordinarily rejected and ridiculed at first. The developer of quantum theory, Max Planck, observed in his autobiography that "a new scientific truth does not triumph by convincing its opponents and making them see the light, but rather because its opponents eventually die, and a new generation grows up that is familiar with it."[2]

RESOLVING AMBIVALENCE

If the cost of indecision is too high, a different approach to ambivalence is to "take arms against a sea of troubles,"[3] seeking to resolve it. The essence of this response is to consider and choose among the available options and take action. As discussed in Chapter 8, such deciding comes easier for some people than for others. It is also more challenging when the stakes are high, with important pros and cons on each side of the dilemma, or when the action would be contrary to the views of significant or powerful others (as in the case of Francis of Assisi).

Something that arises when choosing which way to go at a fork in the road is concern about possible regret later. This phenomenon is familiar as buyer's remorse, but it applies more generally when decisions are made in the face of ambivalence. "Did I do the right thing?" In advance of deciding, this tends to be a stronger concern for perceiving than for judging types of people (Chapter 8). As we shall see in Chapter 11, there are also psychological strategies to reduce regret once a decision has been made.

To resolve ambivalence, there are two basic ways of proceeding, two methods for considering information. The first is called *unbiased processing,* giving systematic open and fair consideration to both (or all) possible paths at a fork in the road. This is what we hope judges and juries do when hearing cases in court—hear and consider all of the evidence on both sides without preexisting bias and reach a fair decision. This requires some time and effort. In Chapter 11 you can try out a method for doing exactly this when resolving ambivalence.

Often, though, you enter into ambivalence with some conscious or unconscious bias. It arises from your own experience and can be influenced by others as well (Chapter 5). Such bias inclines you to take one road rather than another. What often happens in this case is called *biased systematic processing,* "selectively focusing on one side of the issue and tipping the evaluative balance."[4] Even a slight value bias may prompt you to process information in its favor. The confirmation bias described above in avoiding ambivalence can also be used to favor a particular choice in resolving it, paying selective attention to evidence that defends it, perhaps being less critical in evaluating the reliability of sources.

Response amplification takes this defensive strategy a step farther. The pattern here is to resolve ambivalence through extreme commitment to one side of a dilemma. Sigmund Freud described a defense mechanism of *reaction formation* in which people overcompensate in an opposite way. For example, someone who resents having to care for a relative may become overly affectionate and protective. Resolute proponents of antigay legislation periodically turn out to be privately gay themselves. Particularly strident argument may even be motivated by lurking doubts about one's position or knowledge of its falsity. In response amplification it is as if we seek to convince ourselves (and others) that only one of the Janus faces of ambivalence is reality.

Such "protesting too much" is not necessarily a bad thing. New converts can be deeply committed believers, finding fresh meaning that shifts personal identity and restructures their lives.[5] A good example is engagement in Alcoholics Anonymous, which "meets recovering persons at many of their points of need and provides community, behavioral, emotional, and spiritual disciplines" to help them transition, sometimes suddenly, from a self-destructive lifestyle into personal transformation.[6] The early one-and-only-truth fervor of such rebirth can morph over time to internalization of a new program for living.[7] Sometimes such transformation seems to happen spontaneously.[8] A shortcut for biased resolution of ambivalence is to accept the opinion of an authority, reference group, or information source with unambiguous views. When serving as an expert witness in court I found that attorneys who retained me definitely preferred for me to have unequivocal opinions. My tendency as a scientist to acknowledge alternative possibilities led to a short career in forensic psychology.

Whenever you receive information that is inconsistent with your current beliefs or opinions, you have a choice. You can dismiss it or you can choose to be interested and explore it further. I once overheard a predoctoral student talking with her senior advisor in the hallway just outside my faculty office. She had completed a study testing a theory of his and was explaining that her data did not confirm his predictions. "Then you did it wrong," he replied. "Do it over." In my own research I often did not find what I expected, and some of the most important discoveries came from following up on those unpredicted results. Curiosity is the appropriate scientific response to surprise.

Explanation continues to evolve after a decision has been made. There is a human tendency to defend your decision *particularly* when it was an ambivalent choice. This reinterpreting is reflected not only in what you say but also in how you think after the fact. A familiar theme is *sour grapes:* disparagement of the rejected choice. "I wouldn't have enjoyed it anyhow." If you have acted negatively toward or harmed someone, even unintentionally, there is a risk of denigrating or devaluing the person to diminish ambivalent (guilt) feelings.[9] The often-unconscious defensive reasoning is "If I was unkind, then they must have deserved it." Such post-hoc justification of actions can work in both directions: When you act with kindness toward people, your opinion of them tends to improve. Actions drive attitudes, and vice versa. How very far we can go in rationalizing our behavior and beliefs!

Post-hoc justification for a decision can continue to be elaborated and amplified over time. A decision to commit an illegal act may be rationalized, even generalized, into an antisocial identity.[10] Explanations can also emerge from perceiving a pattern in ambiguity, much like Hermann Rorschach's test in which people project form onto random inkblots.[11] It can be comforting to see order in randomness or failure.[12] Orderly explanation is a possible appeal of conspiracy theories.[13]

THE TRAP OF BINARY THINKING

The Zen master holds a stick above a student's head. "If you tell me this is a stick, I will hit you. If you tell me that this is not a stick, I will hit you. If you say nothing, I will hit you." Novices get trapped in either/or thinking and are likely to be rapped on the head. An insightful few respond by reaching up to take the stick, which the master gently releases.

For whatever reason, our human brains are prone to dualistic either/or thinking. Though life is rich in diversity, there is an appealing simplicity to binary perception, the illusion of only two possibilities. We may think of nature as consisting of people versus everything else. Humankind, like nature more generally, is incredibly diverse, but we tend to envision in binary terms: us and them, winner or loser, black and white, friend or enemy, male and female, liberal or conservative. Such dualistic thinking further suggests comparison and competition, which in turn is an invitation for taking sides and for domination. Zen koans like the one above are lessons—sometimes questions or stories—intended to help learners escape from dualism and awaken to a new way of seeing and being in the world.

Seemingly solid categories (the literal meaning of *stereotype*) are seldom uniform. There is wide variability *within* a racial group, biological gender, or political party. Sometimes differences within groups are greater than those between groups. People identified as "conservatives" vary widely in their combinations of beliefs and behavior, as do "liberals." Allegedly different or opposite groups also have much in common. Stereotyping a racial, political, or religious group as all being alike is a mental illusion. People are complex and hold a wide variety of views and values.

Most dichotomous categories are not binary, falling neatly into two clearly separate groups. In apartheid South Africa and during slavery in the United States, elaborate measurement systems were devised to define exactly whether people were Black or White. Different facial features actually vary along a continuum, and arbitrary cutoff points were constructed to reduce diversity into two categories. Consider masculinity and femininity. This once seemed a clear dichotomy, and then along came expanding acronyms like

LGBTQIAPK. As a personality factor, masculinity versus femininity might be thought of as a single dimension ranging from superman to supermodel. Yet masculinity and femininity can be measured as separate personality dimensions; a person can be high on one and low on the other (sex-role stereotyped), high on both (androgynous), low on both (undifferentiated), or any combination.[14] In one study, after transformational experiences, the values of both men and women moved away from sex-role stereotypes to become more similar.[15]

If you felt discomfort arising within you while you were reading the preceding paragraphs, it illustrates an appeal of binary thinking. You may feel inclined to snap back to "No! There are really only two kinds of people." Something in us loves to perceive and take sides, whether in sports, games, debates, wars, or politics. We enjoy choosing up and belonging to a team, an in-group, a tribe. It is beautifully simple. Some people are in; others are out. Someone wins, and someone else loses.

This can be a challenge when counseling distressed couples, who often come to a therapist as if they were going to court to determine which one is at fault, who is in the wrong. It is the stuff of televised entertainment therapy or an advice column, where a guru dispenses "right" answers. A competent marital/family therapist does not take sides; the "client" is not one or both individuals but their *relationship*.

As mentioned in Chapter 5, when two people are ambivalent together, they sometimes take up sides themselves. Each voices the arguments on one side of a question about which both are actually ambivalent. This can occur inadvertently, as they express the poles of their dilemma while trying to resolve it. One speaks for one side, and the other naturally replies with "yes, but. . . . " There is even something appealing about this division of labor; you can watch what is internal ambivalence being acted out as in a debate, and who happens to take up which side of the argument can be arbitrary. However, the act of defending a position does tend to strengthen your commitment to it, and so what was initially an ambivalent topic can become polarized. If one partner then begins to concede the debate, the other may become ambivalent again and even take up the opposite side.

The same can happen at a social level, with groups. Political parties have been known to reverse positions on an issue when conditions change. When one group begins advocating on a topic, another group may reflexively take up the opposite argument, with each becoming ever more committed through public statements. This dance of opposition also has its mental appeal. When there are only two sides, your binary brain tends to perceive them as opposed—right versus wrong, good versus evil—and once that is established, there is no doubt about which one is the side of the angels: your own.

As this dynamic emerges and positions become established, *univalence* can set in on both sides for individuals or groups. Open-minded consideration of relative merits gives way to single-minded allegiance. Such single-mindedness can be viewed as praiseworthy (uncompromising, persevering, stalwart), although the very same behavior can also be labeled as obstinate, inflexible, or pigheaded (see Chapter 5). Unlike ambivalence, univalence is associated with high certainty and quick responses and is prone to hyperbole. Friends are tremendous and foes are horrible.

Perspectives can become still more entrenched when one side (person or group) is isolated from the other. Such segregation—having only similar and like-minded associates—can make extremity seem normal. It happens with alcohol use. As people's drinking increases, they migrate toward heavier-drinking companions and situations. We once offered a free "drinker's check-up" for people who wondered whether their drinking might be harming them.[16] Many drinkers took us up on it. One component of the check-up compared the person's own alcohol use with national survey norms by calculating a percentile: "Out of 100 American men (or women) on average, how many drink less than you do?" Most people who came (voluntarily) for a check-up regarded themselves to be fairly normal drinkers but actually scored around the 98th percentile. They were incredulous—"But *everybody* drinks like I do—some of them even more than I do!" they said—and among their regular associates, it was true.

Geographic separation can have a similar effect. At two universities I attended, the offices of clinical psychology faculty were physically isolated from the rest of the department—on a separate floor or in a different building. Both departments suffered destructive internecine conflicts between clinical and other faculty. Isolation from diversity can foster warring camps. Having an aisle that separates legislators who are from different parties favors polarization, particularly if they never cross the aisle. This kind of segregation can begin early, as with school students forming cliques that include or exclude individuals based on perceived characteristics.

Social media can similarly promote segregation and isolation. Algorithms to promote use of a particular medium tend to feed users more of what they already view and offer more extreme and focused versions. This favors polarization of views as well as the rapid proliferation of confirmatory disinformation and conspiracy theories.

You are not limited or condemned to binary thinking. The

human race is slowly growing past it.[17] When you find yourself walling reality into two categories, take a deep breath and reconsider.[18] People, relationships, emotions, and life quality range far beyond two possibilities. I think of this when someone asks me, "How are you?" The reflexive polite answer is "Fine, and how are you?" In U.S. culture it has become a superficial greeting, not a genuine invitation for intimate self-disclosure. I did have one uncommonly intuitive and unsettlingly honest psychologist friend. If I answered, "Fine," he might say, "I don't think so," and tell me more about my state of mind and heart, just from what he observed in my face and heard in my voice. I don't quite know how he did it, but he was usually right. After a year or so when we met, even passing in the hall, I would say: "Hello Michael! How am I?"

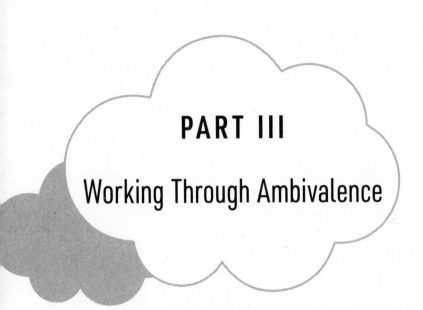

PART III

Working Through Ambivalence

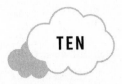

TEN

Getting Clear on Your Values

*If you don't know where you're going,
you might wind up somewhere else.*
—Yogi Berra

In the Danish television drama *Borgen,* the genial Birgitte Nyborg is the leader of a small political party who, through a sequence of unexpected events, becomes the first female prime minister of Denmark. In the first two seasons, acceding first to the time demands of office and then to political advantage, she successively compromises her friends, children, marriage, and her own core values. It doesn't happen all at once; there is no sudden turn to the dark side. It's more like the aphorism that a frog will not jump out of a pot of water if the temperature is gradually increased to boiling.

■ ■ ■

Life's significant choices are often made in the midst of ambivalence. Such decisions gradually shape your life, your character, and your future. Some are made under time pressure. Many are influenced by the situation in which you find yourself and by the people

107

with whom you share it (Chapter 5). Each individual choice may seem small, but they can snowball over time.

Getting clear on what you value most is helpful when facing ambivalent choices. Your decisional balance can be tipped by short-term factors without and within, conscious and unconscious. This chapter invites you to step back and consider what is most important to you, as a context for the daily choices in your life.

WHAT ARE VALUES?

How do you make significant decisions? As discussed in Chapter 4, values are only a part of the directional compass that guides your decisions. Your choices can be tipped by moment-to-moment circumstances, thoughts, emotions, and behaviors. One action then makes the next easier, and there is a certain inertia to habit. At a level deeper than your immediate situation are your beliefs and attitudes that are more stable, but nevertheless evolve over time. Deeper still are the core values that you think of as part of who you *are*. In other words, your choices and actions can be swayed by many factors.

How consistent is what you do and say with the values to which you aspire? In one sense, values can be inferred from your behavior. For example, apart from what you say that you value, how do you actually spend your time and money? What might someone conclude about your values by examining your bank statements or calendar? Actions do speak louder than words.

Is it really meaningful, then, to talk about values apart from what you actually do? Yes, I believe it is. The person you are now is not a finished product. Values are reflected in your goals, hopes, and aspirations, in what you wish to do and become, and in how you understand the meaning and purpose of your life. They represent what you hope to move toward or away from in life. Core values are your enduring convictions about what is right, good, desirable, and worthy. They are a creed, code, or ideal by which you live, the standards against which you evaluate yourself and others.

Getting clearer about what you most value can help you consider how your life might better reflect those values. Without conscious attention and intention, your core values may be overrun by short-term concerns. The noisy immediate influences of the world around you can drown out your own good sense and the softer voices of what matters most.

A starting point is to consider the person you actually are (or at least believe you are) here and now. Here's an interesting experience you could try. List 10 important aspects of yourself, the roles or characteristics that most describe who you are. Only 10, please, so narrow it down from a potentially longer list. You could write them on 10 index cards, sticky notes, or slips of paper, making it easier to move them around in the remaining steps. Next, arrange the list in order, placing at the top the one aspect that *most* defines who you are as a person. They are all important, but which is *most* important? Arrange all 10, from most to least vital aspects of your current self. Finally, a challenging but interesting last step. How many items could you let go of, cross off or remove from the bottom of the list, and still be who you *are*?

Why is this last step difficult? Something in us wants to protect who we believe we are. It is our *identity,* our self-understanding, the story we tell ourselves about ourselves. When someone challenges your self-concept or criticizes you as a person, the natural response is defensive.

WHO ARE YOUR POSSIBLE SELVES?

The person you are now is not necessarily who you will be. It is true that the best guess about what someone will be like at age 80 is what he or she was like at 40. Lifelong kindly people don't normally become mean elders. Yet people do change and grow over time. There seems to be a natural tendency toward self-actualization, to grow into your positive potential, just as an acorn naturally develops into an oak tree with its own knots and gnarls.

One way of thinking about values is as *possible selves,* your ideas about what you might be or become.[1] Possible selves are different from your actual here-and-now self and represent potential futures. Possible selves are, in essence, alternative future versions of yourself. I will briefly discuss five different possible selves that have been described in psychological literature on the subject: your ideal, dream, probable, nightmare, and shadow self.

Ideal Self

One possible self that was explored earliest in psychology is the *ideal* self, the person you believe you ought to be or become. This is not necessarily being like someone else, although the concept of your ideal self may be influenced by people you admire. There is a direct tie here to your core values. If you were the ideal version of yourself, how would you be different? What do you hope to grow *toward* in your life?

The psychologist Carl Rogers was interested in the discrepancy between a person's ideal self and his or her actual experience.[2] He was concerned that people's concept of ideal self is often imposed and internalized from external sources and may be quite at variance with who they really are.[3] If so, significant portions of what you actually experience can become unacceptable in comparison to the ideal self. Rogers believed that mental illness arises from the discrepancy between ideal and actual self—the larger the gap, the greater the suffering. He developed a person-centered form of counseling designed to help people experience and accept who they are.

From this perspective, the healthiest people would be those whose ideal self is identical to their actual self—no discrepancy at all between who they are and who they aspire to be. Would that be mental health or a personality disorder? Narcissistic individuals, for example, have a grandiose sense of self-importance and superiority and tend to see themselves as ideal. Striving toward ideals beyond your current attainment is an honored attribute in many human endeavors, including athletics, art, music, religion, and education.

So what are ideals toward which you hope to grow? These need not be imposed goals. Rather, how would you really choose to be? What is the beacon toward which you steer in your life? That is your ideal self.

Dream Self

Then there is your *dream* self—what you might fantasize about being or becoming.[4] Realism doesn't reign here. Perhaps you romanticize being rich, famous, loved, strong, attractive, or powerful. These are common themes in advertising—fanciful messages about what you should or could be. For example, a young friend of mine is considering buying a roadless forested plot of land in rural Alaska, with a dream of building a log cabin for his family and living off the land. Social groups, organizations, or cultures can promote particular dreams and may even use intentional strategies to break down people's current sense of what is important and meaningful, replacing it with institutional goals and values.[5] Such dreams are the carrot dangling from the end of the stick and may inspire amazing persistence.[6]

Probable Self

In contrast to the dream self, a third possible self is what you imagine is realistic and likely for you. It is what you *expect* to be or become. What would be your best guess as to how you will probably be different (if at all) 5 or 10 years from now?

The probable self can be self-perpetuating. I am personally grateful for mentors who brought out in me capabilities that I did not see in myself. They gently taught me, "Yes, you can." Walter McIver was a charismatic music professor and choirmaster at Lycoming College. I was a psychology major who just enjoyed listening to music, but responding to his invitation to try out for the college choir, I nervously ventured into his office. He greeted me warmly, sat down at the keyboard of his grand piano, and struck a low note. "Sing this note for me like this: A-O-A-O-A." I did my best, and he gradually moved up the keyboard until at last my throat closed up and I said that was all I could do. "Oh my, no!" he replied. "I *like* what I hear, and there is much more there in you. Did you know that you are a first tenor?" And in the months that followed, he gave me a gift that has lasted a lifetime. My probable self expanded a bit that day.

Such influence can also lead in a dark direction. A handsome African American adolescent named Malcolm Little had a life-changing moment when he confided to his high school English teacher that he planned to become an attorney.[7] The White teacher responded that being a lawyer was an unrealistic goal for someone with his skin color and he should be thinking about something that he *could* be. His probable self collapsed. "It was then I began to change inside," he later reported. He started pulling away from White people. He abandoned his dream of becoming an attorney, dropped out of school, and began a life of crime. He was arrested and sentenced to 10 years in prison, where his nickname was Satan. But the story doesn't end there. On release, Mr. Little became a minister who founded several new congregations and proved to be a powerful public speaker. He changed his name to Malcolm X, married and had six daughters, and would visit many nations advocating for racial justice.

Nightmare Self

A fourth possible self is the nightmare self: that which you are afraid you *might* be or become. Beyond what you hope, dream, or expect to be, there are also glimmers of what you fear becoming. A common nightmare self among high-achieving students is the impostor syndrome. For graduate students, it is the fear that somehow you managed to fake your way in but really don't deserve to be there, and if anyone ever discovers how incompetent you really are, you will be cast into outer darkness. In relationships, it can be the fear that if your loved one ever finds out who you really are, you will be unlovable. Nightmare-self themes include poverty, abandonment, failure, shame, and rejection. This is the self from which you run.

Shadow Self

Although it is easily confused with the nightmare self, the shadow self is different in an important way. The nightmare self is what you fear becoming. Potentially even more frightening, the shadow self is what you already *are* but do not recognize. In fact, you are convinced that this is definitely *not* you. The Swiss psychiatrist Carl Jung coined the term "the shadow" to describe unintegrated aspects of personality that are disavowed.[8] They are blind spots, dark and unacceptable corners of the self. Ironically, although you are unaware of your shadow, it is often quite apparent to others. Your shadow can be outed in projection—seeing and responding strongly to the same attribute in other people. It can also pop up in impulsively saying or doing things that may surprise or shock you. Did I say that out loud? Was that really me?[9] A therapeutic goal is to recognize, accept, and integrate these sequestered parts of the self.

INTEGRITY: WHO ARE YOU REALLY?

Now with all of these possible selves roaming around inside, you can just imagine the possibilities for ambivalence. People have multiple values that are often inconsistent and not well organized or integrated.[10] Which values happen to come to the fore may depend on the situation, causing people to manufacture beliefs and reactions on the spot and creating a somewhat fluid sense of identity. In daily life as usual, it is easy to be mostly unconscious of inconsistencies among your own beliefs, attitudes, values, and actions or of conflicts with the expectations of others. If someone gently points out such personal inconsistency, as Professor Rokeach did with his students (see Chapter 4), it can get your attention and prompt change.

As a new assistant professor, I had five years to demonstrate my value to the university within an "up or out" tenure system, so I put my head down and focused on doing good work, using even small blocks of unscheduled time to get tasks done. In anonymous written evaluations after two years, senior faculty critiqued me for being self-centered and uncommitted to the department. It took me by surprise. I had not been going out for coffee or lunch with colleagues or stopping by their offices just to chat, which was a departmental norm. I had to adjust my time priorities somewhat to develop more collegial relationships, which are also important.

This kind of prioritizing is important within your own values. You are constantly choosing how to spend limited resources of time, money, and energy. To what extent are these decisions serving your larger values and longer-term life goals? In Shakespeare's *Hamlet,* Polonius offers this sage advice: "This above all, to thine own self be true."[11] He is talking about *integrity*—living in a way that is consistent with your own core values.[12] People whose lives are well aligned with their personal values tend to be more creative and empathic, have more positive moods, and experience greater meaning in life.[13] On the other hand, those whose lives are discordant with their personal values or serve inconsistent goals are more likely to experience depression, anxiety, anger, and physical symptoms.[14]

WHAT MATTERS MOST TO YOU?

So what are your goals for *being*? What are the values that you want to pursue with the finite time and resources of your life? The box on pages 117–121 contains a varied list of 100 such values that different people might choose.[15] There are different ways to consider your value priorities. Perhaps the simplest is to read through the list and choose the top 5 or 10 that are most important to you. The same set of values is also available online in a format that can be printed out on small cards, with one value per card.[16] In this way you can sort the cards into piles as not important, somewhat important, important, very important, or most important. This can be an interesting process in that it helps you consider what are least and most important guiding values for you. If there are other values that are important to you and not mentioned, you can add them to the list or cards.

Your chosen values at present may be quite different than they were earlier in your life. It is normal for value priorities to change over the years. Sometimes a significant life event causes major rearrangement, even reversal of core values.[17] At this point in your life, however, what are your most important guiding values?

After you have identified your core values (whatever number of values you choose, but not more than 10), here are some questions for your own reflection.

- Among the values you have chosen, can you prioritize them in importance? Is there one that you would say is the most important? Which one might be next in importance, and so on?
- Considering each important value on your list, one at a time, in what ways are you currently showing and pursuing this value?
- Why is each of these values important to you? What people, events, or other influences have helped to make this a priority for you?

One Hundred Possible Life Values

1.	Acceptance	To be accepted as I am
2.	Accuracy	To be correct in my opinions and beliefs
3.	Achievement	To have important accomplishments
4.	Adventure	To have new and exciting experiences
5.	Art	To appreciate or express myself in art
6.	Attractiveness	To be physically attractive
7.	Authority	To be in charge of others
8.	Autonomy	To be self-determined and independent
9.	Beauty	To appreciate beauty around me
10.	Belonging	To have a sense of belonging, being part of
11.	Caring	To take care of others
12.	Challenge	To take on difficult tasks and problems
13.	Comfort	To have a pleasant and comfortable life
14.	Commitment	To make enduring, meaningful commitments
15.	Compassion	To feel and act on concern for others
16.	Complexity	To embrace the intricacies of life
17.	Compromise	To be willing to give and take when reaching agreements
18.	Contribution	To make a lasting contribution in the world
19.	Cooperation	To work collaboratively with others
20.	Courage	To be brave and strong in the face of adversity
21.	Courtesy	To be considerate and polite toward others

22.	Creativity	To create new things or ideas
23.	Curiosity	To seek out, experience, and learn new things
24.	Dependability	To be reliable and trustworthy
25.	Diligence	To be thorough and conscientious in whatever I do
26.	Duty	To carry out my duties and obligations
27.	Ecology	To live in harmony with the environment
28.	Excitement	To have a life full of thrills and stimulation
29.	Faithfulness	To be loyal and true in relationships
30.	Fame	To be known and recognized
31.	Family	To have a happy, loving family
32.	Fitness	To be physically fit and strong
33.	Flexibility	To adjust to new circumstances easily
34.	Forgiveness	To be forgiving of others
35.	Freedom	To be free from undue restrictions and limitations
36.	Friendship	To have close, supportive friends
37.	Fun	To play and have fun
38.	Generosity	To give what I have to others
39.	Genuineness	To act in a manner that is true to who I am
40.	God's Will	To seek and obey the will of God
41.	Gratitude	To be thankful and appreciative
42.	Growth	To keep changing and growing

43. Health	To be physically well and healthy
44. Honesty	To be honest and truthful
45. Hope	To maintain a positive and optimistic outlook
46. Humility	To be modest and unassuming
47. Humor	To see the humorous side of myself and the world
48. Imagination	To have dreams and see possibilities
49. Independence	To be free from depending on others
50. Industry	To work hard and well at my life tasks
51. Inner Peace	To experience personal peace
52. Integrity	To live my daily life in a way that is consistent with my values
53. Intelligence	To keep my mind sharp and active
54. Intimacy	To share my innermost experiences with others
55. Justice	To promote fair and equal treatment for all
56. Knowledge	To learn and contribute valuable knowledge
57. Leadership	To inspire and guide others
58. Leisure	To take time to relax and enjoy
59. Loved	To be loved by those close to me
60. Loving	To give love to others
61. Mastery	To be competent in my everyday activities
62. Mindfulness	To live conscious and mindful of the present moment

63. Moderation	To avoid excesses and find a middle ground
64. Monogamy	To have one close, loving relationship
65. Music	To enjoy or express myself in music
66. Nonconformity	To question and challenge authority and norms
67. Novelty	To have a life full of change and variety
68. Nurturance	To encourage and support others
69. Openness	To be open to new experiences, ideas, and options
70. Order	To have a life that is well-ordered and organized
71. Passion	To have deep feelings about ideas, activities, or people
72. Patriotism	To love, serve, and protect my country
73. Pleasure	To feel good
74. Popularity	To be well-liked by many people
75. Power	To have control over others
76. Practicality	To focus on what is practical, prudent, and sensible
77. Protect	To protect and keep safe those I love
78. Provide	To provide for and take care of my family
79. Purpose	To have meaning and direction in my life
80. Rationality	To be guided by reason, logic, and evidence
81. Realism	To see and act realistically and practically

82.	Responsibility	To make and carry out responsible decisions
83.	Risk	To take risks and chances
84.	Romance	To have intense, exciting love in my life
85.	Safety	To be safe and secure
86.	Self-Acceptance	To accept myself as I am
87.	Self-Control	To be disciplined in my own actions
88.	Self-Esteem	To feel good about myself
89.	Self-Knowledge	To have a deep and honest understanding of myself
90.	Service	To be helpful and of service to others
91.	Sexuality	To have an active and satisfying sex life
92.	Simplicity	To live life simply, with minimal needs
93.	Solitude	To have time and space where I can be apart from others
94.	Spirituality	To grow and mature spiritually
95.	Stability	To have a life that stays fairly consistent
96.	Tolerance	To accept and respect those who differ from me
97.	Tradition	To follow respected patterns of the past
98.	Virtue	To live a morally pure and excellent life
99.	Wealth	To have plenty of money
100.	World Peace	To work to promote peace in the world

Other value: _____

Other value: _____

- What proportion of your time and energy is currently devoted to living these values?
- How would other people know that these are your values? If you were accused of having this value, would there be enough public evidence to convict you?
- Pick out one or two values that you would choose to strengthen. What could you do to express this value more fully in your life?

Chapter 11 offers you a practical method for getting the big picture when you are faced with an ambivalent decision. Your core values stand as a background for this picture, a context within which to make your life choices.

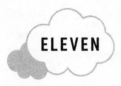

ELEVEN

Getting the Big Picture

Not to decide is to decide.
—Harvey Cox

Aware of it or not, people experiencing ambivalence tend to take one of two broad approaches: to decide or not to decide. As described in Chapter 9, there are many mental machinations for concluding that there really isn't a choice to be made after all or that one side of the apparent dilemma is bogus. Biased systematic thinking can tip the balance without consciously making a decision. Sometimes the mere passage of time without choosing makes the decision for you. That happens, for example, when there is a deadline for deciding, as with Fran's dilemma in Chapter 2 about whether to move to New York for a promotion. To decide or not to decide is an ambivalent dilemma in itself.

Doing the conscious work of deciding—unbiased systematic processing (Chapter 9)—involves stepping back to get the big picture, simultaneously considering all points of view. It's not a new idea. There is an ancient philosophic tradition of laying out all the best arguments on each side of a question, giving them equal and honest consideration.[1] The image of Janus is a fitting metaphor: looking equally in two directions much as a bird, horse, or fish sees simultaneously to the left and the right.

In a letter to his friend Benjamin Franklin in 1772, the chemist and pastor Joseph Priestly lamented how torn he was regarding a difficult career decision before him. It is a classic example of ambivalence, although the word had not yet been invented. Franklin replied by letter with compassionate logic, describing the problem[2]:

> When these difficult cases occur, they are difficult chiefly because while we have them under consideration all the reasons pro and con are not present to the mind at the same time; but sometimes one set present themselves, and at other times another, the first being out of sight. Hence the various purposes or inclinations that alternately prevail, and the uncertainty that perplexes us.

It's a familiar experience, to go back and forth in the mind between the options, first thinking of one and then the other without finding resolution. It is a natural but unhelpful inclination to mull over one perspective at a time. You mentally venture down one path at a fork in the road, pondering its advantages. Later on, you envision another path, with all its attractions and aversions. Perhaps in imagination you wander several times down each branch of the fork or antler, but it brings no resolve. The inner jury hears impassioned arguments from each side and remains undecided. A temporary relief is to stop thinking about it.

Franklin didn't leave it there, however. He continued by describing a method that he used successfully when struggling with ambivalence, which is a good example of unbiased systematic processing:

To get over this, my way is, to divide half a sheet of paper by a line into two columns, writing over the one Pro, and over the other Con. Then during three or four days consideration I put down under the different heads short hints of the different motives that at different times occur to me for or against the measure. When I have thus got them all together in one view, I endeavour to estimate their respective weights; and where I find two, one on each side, that seem equal, I strike them both out: If I find a reason pro equal to some two reasons con, I strike out the three. If I judge some two reasons con equal to some three reasons pro, I strike out the five; and thus proceeding I find at length where the balance lies; and if after a day or two of farther consideration nothing new that is of importance occurs on either side, I come to a determination accordingly. And tho' the weight of reasons cannot be taken with the precision of algebraic quantities, yet when each is thus considered separately and comparatively, and the whole lies before me, I think I can judge better, and am less likely to take a rash step; and in fact I have found great advantage from this kind of equation, in what may be called moral or prudential algebra.

Franklin's logical scientific mind comes through in corresponding with a fellow scientist. Even if this is not how your own mind works, the method has merit, and indeed it became a therapeutic approach for helping people to make difficult decisions, introduced (pleasingly) by a psychologist named Janis.[3] This big-picture method has been around for a long time, and I don't know a better way to arrive at a decision in the midst of ambivalence.

Several aspects of Franklin's method are noteworthy. First, he took his time in putting together his two-column list. He did it over a period of days, as different reasons occurred to him. It is not something to do in a single session. This takes into account what he observed, that the mind tends to go back and forth among different possible paths. Second, he was listing "different motives," which are broader than logical reasons. Feelings, experience, and intuitions are also considered. Here is a good place to consider your own core values (Chapter 10) and how they converge with each possible choice. Third, Franklin assigned subjective *weights* to each of the motives on his lists—how *important* each reason is. He didn't mention assigning numeric values, although one could do so as a way of weighing relative importance. These are *subjective* weights, according to how important they seem to you. Then, in a kind of "moral algebra" or accounting, he began crossing out equivalent and counterbalancing values on both sides to solve the equation.

Whether or not the weighting and canceling steps appeal to you, constructing this kind of *decisional balance* is a helpful way to put together the big picture for your own consideration. You can adapt the method to your own situation. Perhaps there are more than two possible choices. You could list separately the advantages and disadvantages of each choice. An example of this comes later in this chapter. You might run through a list of different possible considerations, such as:

- Short-term consequences
- Longer-term consequences
- Your core values
- Emotional factors
- Financial considerations
- Impact on loved ones
- Impact on the community
- Consistency with your core values (Chapter 10)
- Moral or spiritual considerations
- Legal implications
- Intuition or hunch
- Past experience

How you do it is up to you. The point is to take your time and construct as large a list of considerations as you can, giving equal consideration to all possible paths. Even seemingly silly considerations can be included. If it occurs to you, write it down.

The simplest form is the two-column method described by Franklin. An often-used decisional balance format retains the two columns, but lists in separate rows the pros and cons, the advantages and disadvantages for each column. This creates a 2-by-2 table that looks like this:

	Option 1	Option 2
Pros or advantages		
Cons or disadvantages		

Often the choice is between making a change and maintaining the status quo—keeping things as they are. The table might look like this for a current smoker:

	Stop smoking	Continue smoking
Pros or advantages	Reduce long-term health risk Save money Set good example for my kids Not be a slave to nicotine Breathe better Taste food more?	No withdrawal discomfort Helps me relax I have a right to smoke

	Stop smoking	Continue smoking
Cons or disadvantages	Nicotine withdrawal Feeling deprived Feeling tense	Social disapproval Cost of cigarettes Limits my dating options

Notice that the same motive can appear in the diagonal cells, in both the advantages of one option and the disadvantages of the other. Saving money is among the advantages of stopping smoking, and the ongoing cost of cigarettes is a disadvantage of continuing to smoke. That's OK. In fact, every advantage in one column may have a corresponding disadvantage in the other, particularly when the columns are opposites as to change or not to change.

The options are not always opposites. A Go-Go candy store decision (Chapter 2) can be between two similarly attractive alternatives. In this case there may be no significant disadvantages of either choice. On the other hand, a No-No trap (lesser of two evils) decision will have disadvantages on both sides and may or may not involve positive advantages. In the yoyo (Go-No) type of ambivalence, you are weighing the pros and cons of a single option, so there may be only those two cells. The four-cell decisional balance is clearest with the pendulum type of ambivalence, in which there are advantages (Go) and disadvantages (No) on both sides in the choice between two options. Use whatever kind of box makes the most sense to you in a particular case.

There can also be more than two branches at a fork in the road. In choosing a treatment for cancer, the decision may be among multiple options, each with evidence of effectiveness as well as unpleasant effects or risks. The basic decisional balance method can still be used, and it's far easier to write it down than to try keeping all of this in mind at the same time.

Here is a real-life example that many individuals or couples face: whether to have a child or children. The table on page 130 has three columns and is one that might be constructed over a period of weeks or months. The options under consideration are pregnancy, adoption, and no children. There are still more possible options, of course, such as in vitro fertilization or a surrogate mother. For illustration purposes, consider just those three. The illustrative entries in each cell are hypothetical and are not meant to be generally applicable.

Notice that the lists are longer in some boxes than in others, but this in itself is not decisive. An item in a shorter-list box may be disproportionately important and override several other items, as mentioned in Franklin's instructions to his friend. Some items may seem silly or relatively unimportant in the big picture, but they are still in the lists. Two partners making this decision together might have very different lists in each box, and they could keep their balance sheets separate or combine them. It is also possible that an item in one partner's list could be a nonstarter or deal breaker for the other. Obviously ongoing discussion is needed when a decision involves more than one person, and it can also be helpful to talk it over with a neutral or professional third party. The original decisional balance method was intended for such use by a neutral facilitator to help people in making difficult choices without favoring resolution in one direction or the other. It can also be used in leadership and group decision making.[4]

So give it a try! Choose an issue or decision about which you are ambivalent and fill in a decisional balance chart like the ones

A Decisional Balance Chart for Three Options

Having a child by pregnancy	Having a child by adoption	Not having children
Pros or advantages		
A child to love and see grow up	A child to love and see grow up	More freedom with time and money
A special kind of relationship	A special kind of relationship	Less stress
Someone to love so deeply	Someone to love so deeply	Free to volunteer and travel
Unique experience bearing a child	So many children in need of a home	No empty nest when they leave
Carry on the family name	Strengthen our relationship?	Can care for other children
Biological clock is ticking	A lifelong friend	
We *want* a child of our own	Tax deduction	
Strengthen our relationship?		
A lifelong friend		
Tax deduction		
Cons or disadvantages		
Huge life and time commitment	Huge life and time commitment	Many missed unique experiences
Huge financial commitment	Huge financial commitment	Would we regret this choice later?
What ifs, unknowns	Effect on careers?	No one to care for us in old age?
Negative effect on careers?	What ifs, unknowns	No one to give inheritance
Create a new life? Others in need	Probably can't get an infant	
	Uncertain genes and history	
	Relationship with birth parents?	
	Child abuse and trauma?	

shown above. It doesn't have to be a major dilemma; you can prac-tice this with smaller choices. Your chart might have only two boxes, like the relative attractions in a Go-Go situation or comparing the adversities in a No-No conflict. It might have four boxes like the smoker's example above, listing the pros and cons of two different choices, or even more, as in the three-option example about chil-dren. You can take your time filling in the boxes; it doesn't have to be done all in one day. It may also be helpful to talk over the options with someone who listens well.

WEIGHING OPTIONS

It often happens that when seeing the big picture, the choice seems clear, or at least clearer. This was an early surprise in research with motivational interviewing (MI), which helps people explore their own reasons for change. In the early 1980s I was thinking of MI just as a preparation for treatment of alcohol use disorders,[5] something like priming the pump to get people ready and willing to accept professional help. In an early study my colleagues and I randomly assigned problem drinkers to receive a session of MI immediately (the drinker's check-up mentioned in Chapter 9) or to be on a wait-ing list to receive the same thing later.[6] After the MI session we gave everyone a list of local programs where they could be treated for problematic alcohol use. We predicted that compared to those on the waiting list, people receiving MI would be more likely to seek specialist treatment. We were wrong. In fact, almost no one went for treatment, but those in the MI group showed a large immedi-ate reduction in their drinking, whereas people on the waiting list showed no apparent change until they were later offered MI. Once they got over the motivational hump of seeing a need for change, they went ahead and did it on their own. Many studies have now shown an effect from this kind of brief counseling for a variety of health concerns.[7] Making the decision itself can be a big head start.

Sometimes going through a decisional balance process is not enough in itself. One path may appear to be the best choice, but *can* you do it? A smoker, for example, might believe that it's really important to quit yet doubt that it's possible. Some additional help or resources beyond those discussed in this book may be needed to do what seems the right thing. In addition to professional assistance, evidence-based advice on a wide variety of issues can be found in self-help books and online. Unfortunately, many kinds of self-help advice have little or no scientific basis, and there is little help for consumers in evaluating the validity of what is offered, so be cautious. Some books and websites do specify the evidence for the approaches that they describe. You can also ask health professionals for recommendations of self-help resources.

But what if getting the big picture in itself doesn't point to a clear choice? What if all the reasons in your columns balance each other out in Franklin's moral algebra? Sometimes the poles of ambivalence really are evenly balanced. It can be useful to confide in several trustworthy friends or family members and talk over your options, listening for additional considerations. Perhaps there is further information that would help in tipping the balance. You can discuss your dilemma with a professional who has relevant expertise. If there is no need for a rapid decision, then some additional time for reflection may help with clarity. Sometimes it is possible to try a step or two down one path without committing to the whole distance.

And sometimes you just have to make a choice and live with it.

The way forward then is to reach a decision and follow that path. It might even seem to be an arbitrary choice. It may not become clear for some time how it will go or even if there was one single right path. It could turn out in the long run that it wasn't the best choice. The alternative is to remain encamped at the fork in the road.

REGRET

It is possible, of course, that when you make a decision and follow through with it, you will regret it later. For some people, in fact, avoiding subsequent regret is a prime consideration when making decisions in the first place.[8]

Like ambivalence, regret is a common human experience, and there is much theory and research on the subject.[9] So what is it? Regret is the nasty feeling that you can experience when you realize or imagine that things would be better if only you had made a different decision. It has two necessary components.[10] The first is disappointment, comparing your current situation with how you believe things would be if you had decided differently. Add to that some self-blame or guilt for having made the wrong decision, and you've got the experience of regret.

Because regret is so common, people have developed a broad array of ways to react when they feel it.[11] Like responses to ambivalence itself (Chapter 9), responses to regret tend to fall into two broad categories. The first approach is cognitive, mainly designed to avoid or reduce the unpleasant emotion associated with regret. You might find justifications for the decision you made, that it really was the best choice after all. Perhaps there is a silver lining to what you decided; these often begin with the words "at least. . . ." If you took time to give careful consideration to the possible options in light of your values, you can take comfort that it was a reasonable choice given all that you knew at the time. You could devalue what you didn't choose, deciding that it would not have been all that good, or that you really didn't want it anyhow. You could deny personal responsibility for having made the choice: Someone else decided or persuaded you to do it.

The other broad approach to regret is to do something about it. Sometimes the decision can be undone or reversed. You can accept and express your regret, perhaps in the form of an apology to anyone who was harmed by your choice, and do what you can to make it right. This is the heart of restorative justice.[12] You can adjust your future actions in light of what you learned so that further decisions have better results.

Making a decision, the focus of this chapter, is a good beginning. Once you have made a choice, how can you get and keep yourself moving down that path? Sometimes having made the decision is enough in itself, and off you go. It may also take a bit more motivational work to launch you on your way. That is the topic of Chapter 12.

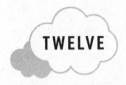

TWELVE

Getting Out of the Woods

I took the [road] less traveled by, and that has made all the difference.
—Robert Frost, *The Road Not Taken*

You didn't intend to get lost in the deep forest, but it happened. Fortunately, you came prepared. You brought along a sleeping bag and small packing tent that kept you warm and dry last night, and this morning you were able to build a small fire. You wore appropriate clothing and shoes and have enough food and water for another day or two. What you don't have is a compass. If only you were in Iceland, it would be easy: The local joke is that if you are lost in an Icelandic forest, just stand up (because the trees are short). You know that this is a sizable forest, and the treetop canopy obstructs your view of the sun by day and the stars by night. There are no trails or stream to follow, and in exploring last night before it grew dark, you discovered that you had been wandering in circles.

Now it's a new day, and you want to get out of the trees. You know from a map that the forest is not more than six or seven miles on a side. You're not sure which direction to head, but you reason that if you could just walk in a straight line in any direction, you would eventually find your way out. But how to do that—how to keep from retracing your steps and walking around in circles again?

Aha! You have an idea. You find a tree that is some distance away from you, and looking past it you focus on a second tree that is farther away. Then keeping those two trees in your line of sight, you spot yet a third tree still farther away that lies in a straight line with the other two. Now you walk from tree 1 to tree 2, keeping an eye on tree 3. As you approach tree 2, you then spot a fourth tree in a straight line out beyond tree 3, and so on. In this way, with any luck, you can keep moving from tree to tree in a reasonably straight line and eventually find your way to a road or stream or to the forest's edge.

■ ■ ■

Getting unstuck from ambivalence is a bit like that. A natural tendency is to keep going around in circles, thinking first about one possibility and then another, retracing your steps. Another possibility is to find a way to be comfortable living with ambivalence (Chapter 13). To get out of the forest, however, you would pick a direction and keep moving that way. This can feel uncomfortable at first. Particularly with the yoyo and pendulum types of ambivalence, moving in one direction can give you second thoughts. To avoid more nights in the forest, though, you would just keep on moving in a straight line, undeterred by second thoughts, from tree to tree to tree.

Reaching a decision is a first step in resolving ambivalence. That was the focus of Chapter 11. Carrying out that decision can be a longer process of putting your choice into action and coming to peace with your decision.

THINKING AND TALKING YOUR WAY OUT

The interior work of resolving ambivalence has to do with what you say to yourself (in silent thoughts, writing, or even aloud) and to other people about your choice. You are literally talking yourself through the process. George Carlin observed that "the reason I talk to myself is because I'm the only one whose answers I accept." It's true enough. In your own talk you are, in essence, discovering, rehearsing, and strengthening your motivation to keep on moving.

Several types of language are useful here. You are already familiar with these forms of speech. Whenever you make a request of someone, you listen carefully to what they say in response. Why do you do that? Because what they say gives you clues about whether or not it will happen.[1] Suppose, for example, that you ask a friend to do something for you. The specific content of the request doesn't matter here, because the types of language that you will be listening for are the same. Here are some things that your friend might say in reply to your request:

- I would like to do that for you (and then you listen for a "but . . . ").
- I wish I could do that for you.
- I might be able to do it.
- I could do it.
- I can do it.
- I should do it.
- I know it's important to you.
- I'm willing to do it.
- I'm going to do it.

Can you feel the differences among these? Some of them sound hopeful, others not so much. This is the language of change, a negotiating dance of words that happens when people make and respond to requests.[2] By living in society, you already know this dance, although you may not have thought about the specific steps. The same kinds of language are used when making requests. For example:

- Would you like to . . .
- Could you . . .
- Are you willing to . . .
- Will you . . .

Below are seven specific types of self-motivational language that were discussed in Chapter 3. These were clarified through decades of research on listening to what people said during counseling to help them make changes.[3] We found that such speech does in fact predict later behavior.[4] It's possible to be dishonest, of course, as when people say things they don't mean. But when people talk honestly about themselves, these kinds of language can strengthen their motivation for change.[5]

You can practice these for yourself if you wish. Start with a still-ambivalent topic on which you have decided the direction in which you want or choose to move. You can generate each type of change talk about the direction you choose. These are things that you could say to yourself or to someone else, but I suggest first that you actually write them down. On a tablet or sheet of paper, write at the top the decision that you made (perhaps in Chapter 11). The tasks in this chapter may not make much sense unless you are thinking of something specific that you want or have decided to do. Then try out these seven different kinds of statements.

To show specific examples of each kind of change talk, I will offer some of my own self-talk as I worked through ambivalence about exercising when I was first diagnosed with "pre-diabetes." I knew, of course, that regular activity is one of the best things you can do to stay strong and healthy as you age, particularly if you are in a fairly sedentary occupation like mine. I had plenty of excuses *not* to exercise, and I don't need to go into those here. Being diagnosed was a good motivation to give it more serious consideration, although many people with diabetes (or other chronic illnesses) still don't do what they need to do to be healthy.[6] Even having a heart attack may not be enough to persuade people to stop smoking and change their diet and physical activity. So how might I talk myself into doing the right stuff to stay healthy? As I offer examples, you can come up with your own statements on the ambivalent topic of your choice. Don't just think about it. Write them down!

Desire

Desire language is basically a way of saying "I want." A *desire* statement might start with the words *I want to, I wish to, I would enjoy,* or *I would like to.* Here are some of mine.

- I would *like* to keep my eyesight.
- I *look forward* to playing with my grandchildren.
- I do *enjoy* some kinds of physical activity.
- I *want* to do what it takes to stay healthy.

What desire statements might you make about your own chosen direction? Try writing some down using starter words for desire: *want, wish, like, enjoy.*

Ability

A different form of speech is *ability* language, which says it's possible for you. Ability statements might begin with *I can, I could, I am able to,* or *I know how to.*

- I have always liked bicycling, and I guess I *could* do more of that.
- It's *possible* for me to get some exercise equipment to use at home.
- I think I'd be *able* to exercise in the morning for an hour or so.
- I probably *can* do that two or three days a week.

What ability statements can you make about the decision you chose? What can or could you do? (The difference between those two words is interesting in itself. Which one feels easier for you to say, and why?) What would be possible; what would you be able to do?

Reasons

Reason statements explain why you would choose as you did. There are two general forms:

- If I do this, then . . . [and you give a positive reason for the choice you made].
- If I don't do this, then . . . [and you state why the path you chose is better than the alternative].

A good start is to come up with three different reasons to do what you choose:

1. The doctor said that *if* I exercise regularly, *then* it will help keep my blood sugar level down.

2. *If* I *do* exercise, I might not need to go on insulin.

3. I remember what the "complications" can be *if* I *don't* control my diabetes, and I definitely don't *want* to go blind or lose my feet. (This statement doubles up reason and desire.)

So what are at least three good reasons supporting the choice you made? Make a list.

Need

Need language emphasizes importance. Some common forms are *I need to, I have to, I must,* and *it is important for me to.* What can you say about the importance of what you chose? You don't have to explain why. In fact, doing so would turn it into a reason (which is also OK).

- I've *got to* start exercising more.
- Exercise is *important* for me.
- I really *must* be more physically active.

Try writing down a few of these. You can add "because . . . " if you wish, doubling up with a reason.

Activating Language

It is possible to want and need, to have good reasons and ability, and yet not be willing or ready. Activating statements are not quite

"I will," but they are getting close. Here are some possible kinds of statements:

- I am ready to ...
- I am willing to ...
- I am prepared to ...
- I plan to ...
- I intend to ...
- I have decided to ...

Regarding exercise, I might have said to myself or others:

- I am *willing to consider* joining a gym.
- I *plan* to exercise for 45 minutes three nights a week.
- I have *decided* that it's important enough to buy some exercise equipment.

So what are you willing, planning, considering, or ready to do? Write down some statements.

Commitment

Commitment speech is stronger still. This is the language used to make promises and enter into agreements. It says what you are *going* to do. If you were asked in court, "Will you tell the truth, the whole truth, and nothing but the truth?", the judge would not accept any of the statements above: *I want to! I could! I have good reasons to! I need to!* or *I am willing to consider it!* The only acceptable answer is *I will.*[7]

Some possible forms of commitment language include *I will, I am going to, I promise,* and *I guarantee.* Restating my readiness statements above, commitment language would be:

- I am *going to* join a gym.
- I *will* exercise for 45 minutes three nights a week.
- I *promise* to buy some exercise equipment.

So what statements of this kind are you prepared to make regarding the choice you made? What do you think you'll do?

Taking Steps

Often by the time people decide to do something, they have already taken some small steps in that direction, as if preparing or trying it out at least mentally. Here are some from my own situation regarding increased physical activity:

- I looked online to see what an elliptical machine would cost
- I bought a pair of comfortable shoes for exercising
- I asked my doctor what kind of activity would be safe for me.

What (if anything) have you already done to consider, prepare for, lean toward, or try out the choice or change you're considering? Even small steps count. If you don't think of any, what steps *could* you take to move in the desired direction?

A CLINICAL EXAMPLE

Sometimes people find it hard to keep moving in one direction on their own. With conflicting motivations, there is a natural tendency to keep switching back and forth among them rather than going from tree to tree in a straight line. We developed the method of motivational interviewing[8] to help guide people out of the woods of ambivalence. Typically a conversation begins with people describing a change they have been considering (or wanting or needing to make), but haven't managed to do so far—in other words, something about which they are ambivalent. While listening to and respecting their hesitancies, the interviewer helps them voice their own motivations for change and keep moving forward. This method has been shown to help people get unstuck with quite a few different types of change.[9] It can help people either increase or decrease behavior. Here is an example interview with Charles, whose concern is the amount of time he is spending on the internet.

INTERVIEWER: Tell me a bit about what's on your mind.

CHARLES: I really enjoy surfing the web, meeting and talking to people there. I'm on for hours every day, and sometimes I think it's too much, but it's just what I do. *A clear statement of ambivalence*

I: There are things that are good about it for you, and also maybe some less good aspects. *Echoing his ambivalence*

C: Well, I'm not sure it's all that good even for me really. I log in and before I know it hours have passed. *Reason for change*

I: It really engages you, maybe too much.

C: Right. I mean it fills in the time for me, but I don't do much else. *Reason*

I: How would you want to spend the time if you weren't on screens?

C: We have two little kids, 2 years and 6 months old, and I like to spend time with them. *Desire*

I: And their mother?

C: Yes, sure. We all live together.

I: What do you enjoy most about your time together?

C: They're growing up so fast, and I think I miss a lot. I want to be there for them. I mean I work all day, so mostly we can be together at night or on the weekend, and that's when I'm mostly on the computer. We like playing with them together when we can. *Reason* *Desire* *Desire*

I: Your family is pretty important to you.

C: They are, and I feel guilty sometimes like I'm not doing my part. *Reason*

I: And what else might you enjoy doing when you're not on the internet?

C: I like dirt biking, and sometimes we go to the zoo or out for food together. That's fun. I have some friends, too, and I don't see them much. *Desire* *Reason*

I: How important would you say it is for you to spend less time online and more doing other things like with your family?

C: How important?

I: Yes. Like on a scale from 0 to 10, how important do you think it is?

C: I don't know. Maybe 7 or 8. *Need*

I: Wow—pretty important then! So what could you do if you did decide to spend more time away from the internet? How might you do that?

C: Maybe I could set a time limit for myself, like just an hour a day. Actually I should probably do that with our 2-year-old as well. When I'm not with him and his mom is busy, he's getting my bad habit and watching TV.   *Ability*

   Reason

I: You think you could stick with a time limit.

C: Sure. I mean it's a big change for me, but I could do it. I could set a timer.   *Ability*

I: Are you willing to do it?

C: Right away?

I: Well, whenever you choose, but is that something you're willing to try?

C: I think it would be a good idea.   *Readiness*

I: And why is that?

C: Like I said, the kids are growing up and I want to be there to see it. I just feel like I'm getting way too hooked by the stuff on the web.   *Reason*

   Reason

I: Hooked. Like it's controlling you.

C: Kind of. There's no end to it really. I just get kind of mindless and the days fly by. When I think about it, I don't like that.   *Reason*

   Desire

I: You're thinking maybe it's time. So what do you think you'll do then?

C: I like the idea of no more than an hour a day.

I: Do you think you can do that?

C: Yeah, I do. Maybe I'll even start tonight.   *Ability*

I: Really. Tonight. It's up to you.

C: Sure, why not? I'll try it.   *Commitment*

I: Makes sense to me!

What the interviewer is doing here may look simple but it is actually quite skillful and takes some practice. The interviewer could have spent more time talking about all the things Charles likes about the internet, why he wouldn't want to change, and the obstacles to doing so. It also would have gone very differently if Charles was being told why and how he should do it. Instead the interviewer asked particular questions and highlighted aspects of what Charles said to help him keep moving out of the forest. Charles was literally talking himself into change. Just as you listen to what people say when you ask them to do something for you, what someone says during an interview like this predicts whether it is going to happen.[10] By the way, we have found that it's not essential to get to commitment language right away for change to happen. All of the kinds of change talk seem to have their own momentum.

Using Your Own Motivational Statements

Could you do that on your own?[11] Actually that's how it happens normally. The statements that you wrote in the previous section before this example were in your own words, and using them can help to strengthen your motivation and commitment to do what you have decided. They can help you keep moving down the path you chose. You could keep your list in a place where you will see it often. You can add to it. You can say the statements quietly to yourself as reminders. You could speak them aloud to others.

Don't expect perfection. You might go three steps forward and two steps back, but keep moving forward. Perfectionism is the main downfall of New Year's resolutions: taking your statement to be a *rule*. Break the rule once and you may abandon your original intention. Instead of giving up, keep renewing your motivations for the choice that you made. Saying your statements aloud to other people can increase your commitment.

ACTING YOUR WAY OUT

Language isn't everything. Actions speak louder than words. You can enact your decision by what you do. Can you break it down into smaller steps and take them one at a time? Not just saying but *doing* things can move you farther down the path that you have chosen.

If the path is really new, your actions at first can feel like, well, acting. Like riding a bicycle, new behavior can feel uncomfortable and awkward at first. That's how you learn many new things. Living as if your choice is already a fact is one way of getting used to it.[12] Going from heavy daily alcohol use to being a nondrinker can be a huge lifestyle change, and the aphorism "Fake it till you make it" contains the wisdom of lived experience.

So in addition to strengthening your motivation by what you say, how about putting your intention into action? Doing so further strengthens your commitment. What steps could you take to move yourself farther down the chosen path? Over time in my own transition to a low-fat, vegetarian way of eating I read books on the subject, stocked up on healthy foods, tried new recipes, learned to use a spiralizer, told friends what I was doing, even bought some new cookware to enjoy.

Steps like that don't have to be done all at once. Implementing a new decision can take time, whether for an individual, a family, an organization, or a nation. As with the tree-to-tree example, once you're out of the woods you can keep an eye on the horizon and continue moving toward it with steps in the right direction.

A FINAL CHAPTER

So you have read this far in this book without succumbing to ambivalence. The journey began with the nature, flavors, and language of ambivalence. Part II explored its sources, influences, unconscious forms, and effects, and then how people respond to ambivalence, including some personality differences. This Part III on working through ambivalence began with exploring your values and getting a big picture as a context for choosing your direction at a fork in the road. This chapter focused on thinking, talking, and acting your way out of the ambivalence forest once you have made a choice. However, as discussed in the opening chapter, ambivalence is not always to be avoided. Janus has important strengths through being able to look in two directions at once, and ambivalence can be advantageous and even enjoyable. Chapter 13 is about living with and embracing ambivalence.

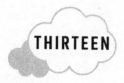

THIRTEEN

Embracing Ambivalence

> *Tempted by simplicity and haunted by complexity, contemporary*
> *[humanity] has the choice of becoming a connoisseur of ambiguity*
> *or becoming paralyzed.*
> —Stephen Shapiro, "The Ambivalent Animal"[1]

Life would not be improved by eradicating ambivalence. Perceiving, considering, and choosing among alternative futures is a remarkable ability and responsibility of humankind and is a defining characteristic of democracies. Life stories great and small are shaped by ambivalence. U.S. presidents and other heads of government face anguished ambivalent decision points and are remembered for the choices they made.

At an individual level, ambivalence raises questions about how you will choose to be, and the decisions you make will in turn shape who you are. The ability to perceive situations from different perspectives is a fundamental element in creativity and in generating new possibilities. Ambivalence is a first step toward change[2] and a necessary step in unlearning inaccurate information and beliefs.[3] It also fosters openness and less selective bias toward new information. Hoping merely to preserve the status quo is a recipe for unhappiness, because change is inevitable.

Ambivalence is also important and valuable at a social level. Dialectic tensions and their resolution lie at the heart of politics and religion.[4] Just as music is enriched by counterpoint, having a diversity of views can foster, and indeed is vital for better decision making in organizations. Abraham Lincoln famously appointed to his cabinet not only allies, but all of his major rivals from the presidential election of 1860. Ambivalent leaders spend more time and consider a variety of perspectives before deciding, whereas unambivalent single-minded leaders may do great harm through impulsive or unreflective action. The public expression of ambivalence (rather than certitude) can motivate new action.[5]

A social corollary is that collective wisdom, which is more likely to contain ambivalence, surpasses individual judgment. In the presbyterian polity that influenced formation of the U.S. constitution, leaders were elected to discern together rather than "lord it over" or simply mirror the views of the governed.[6] Such a process is not about defeating or destroying opposing views. It is about collaborating (literally "working together") and compromising (literally "promising together") through a process of group wisdom that is more than the sum of its individual members' views.

ADAPTING TO CHANGE

Social and technological changes can dramatically affect individuals as well as business and industry. Entire occupations can disappear. Before the emergence of supermarkets, milk was delivered daily door to door in glass bottles. I vividly remember our neighborhood milkman at the door tearfully pleading with my parents not to end their delivery order. With the advent of home refrigeration the iceman no longer cometh, and with the internet, books and sales began migrating to online formats. Music transitioned from vinyl records to cassettes and 8-tracks, then to compact discs and to iTunes. How do businesses respond when such changes occur? Given the human tendency for binary thinking (Chapter 9), CEOs often categorize a particular change as either good or bad and respond accordingly.

But what if an executive is ambivalent, perceiving a change as both good and bad? This question was addressed in a study of 104 German businesses during a major expansion of the European Union (EU) to include former Soviet states.[7] CEOs were asked to rate separately how good the positive aspects were and how bad the negative. Some CEOs were unambivalent, regarding the change to be mostly a good thing; others saw it as primarily a bad thing. Ambivalence was defined as the similarity of a CEO's positive and negative evaluation levels. As it turned out, the companies whose CEOs were ambivalent about EU expansion were the most likely to take adaptive action in response to the change, and their actions were larger in scope, more novel, and entailed greater risk. CEO ambivalence did predict organizational action, but with an important caveat. Remember that ambivalence was defined as having similar levels of perceived good and bad aspects of the change. In this definition, ambivalence would encompass both those who saw very little that was either good or bad, and those who simultaneously perceived more intense positive and negative aspects. The former were essentially indifferent about the EU change, whereas the latter were truly ambivalent in perceiving both significant positive and important negative implications. It was only the latter (those embracing both important pros and cons) who took action to respond to the EU change—more than did companies whose CEOs were indifferent or who saw only good or bad implications. Organizations with ambivalent CEOs considered and implemented a broader range of adaptive strategies, including approaches that were more novel and involved more risk.

ANOTHER WAY

It seems that ambivalence can prompt people to perceive and consider a broader range of possibilities. The dialectic of contradictory perspectives may uncover yet a third way that is neither of the seeming opposites. What I have loved about cross-country skiing is freedom from lifts and groomed trails—the ability to simply head off through the trees, up hills and down, across unbroken snow. It is unbound by predefined paths. The Zen koans mentioned in Chapter 9 engage out-of-the-box thinking that transcends the obvious possibilities.

The path of nonviolent resistance is a classic example of a third way that is neither fight nor flight, domination nor surrender. Often a third way requires not only alternative action, but a different way of seeing and thinking. There is a sudden or gradual "aha" that transforms how reality is perceived. Just as peace is much more than an absence of war, a nonviolent way of being is more than refraining from harming others. It is doing that which is incompatible with harm—actively promoting the well-being of others.

My perspectives as a writer have surely changed over half a century of practice. Early on, I perceived article reviewers as annoying adversaries to be overcome, and I remember having been outraged when an editor altered my language. Yet what is needed to become a better writer (or person, for that matter) is not to reject, but to be open to and learn from critique. I have worked with a dozen different book publishers over the years. Some have published what I sent them with little or no change, which means that what I submit must be a finished product with which I am satisfied. But for two decades now I have preferred to work with the same publisher whenever possible, and I do so precisely because of the quality of editing. A manuscript first goes through a developmental editing process that requires rewrites, and then it goes through copy editing to fix the fine points. Rewrites can require a lot of work, but I now prize rather than resent them. As a result, the books are so much better than my first drafts.

An alternative way that has received increasing attention in psychotherapy is *acceptance*.[8] It is captured succinctly in Reinhold Niebuhr's variously quoted "serenity prayer," penned in the 1930s:

> *God give me the serenity to accept things which cannot be changed;*
> *Give me courage to change things which must be changed;*
> *And the wisdom to distinguish one from the other.*

Some things are conditions to be accepted; don't mistake a condition for a problem. Acceptance is letting go of distress about and efforts to change what is not changeable. Forgiveness is such an act: relinquishing the wish for a different past or for harm to come to an offender.[9] Then there are other things that can be—or in Niebuhr's language, *must* be changed. Deciding which is which does, indeed, require some wise discernment. The dual hazards are in persistently trying to move the unmovable and failing to alter what needs changing.

SYNTHESIS

A classic sequence in philosophy is thesis-antithesis-synthesis. The thesis and antithesis are two seemingly opposite assertions, and a synthesis combines or reconciles them. A common example is that young children tend to look up to their parents as all-knowing and powerful. Adolescence can then bring the antithesis, that parents know nothing and are hopelessly inept. Over time, a more balanced view of and relationship with parents can emerge, a middle way between adulation and rebellion. There is a quip attributed to Mark Twain: "When I was a boy of 14, my father was so ignorant I could hardly stand to have the old man around. But when I got to be 21, I was astonished at how much the old man had learned in seven years." The same transition can apply to attitudes toward authority figures more generally.

The discipline of psychology had its roots in 19th-century philosophy and religion, a heritage that was perfectly natural and comfortable in 1902 for William James,[10] who is often called the father of American psychology. As the 20th century progressed, however, religion was being described as a source of mental illness and immaturity[11] and became a taboo subject for psychological research except within a relatively isolated subspecialty in the psychology of religion.[12] Relative to the clients they served, psychologists as a group were far less religiously oriented.[13] It was as if psychology itself went through an adolescent rebellion. Toward the end of the 20th century, however, the discipline warmed to spirituality and religion, and the American Psychological Association published books on the topic for the first time.[14] It was as if the discipline said, "Perhaps our parents knew something after all!" It became acceptable again to live in both worlds at once.

When new and potentially conflicting information is encountered, how do you incorporate it? One approach is *assimilation,* which modifies the facts to fit within your existing thinking. For example, an intelligent and likable member of a previously disliked group might be considered to be a rare exception to the stereotyped rule. In contrast, *accommodation* requires some change in thinking itself. The "exception" might create ambivalence about the prior stereotype and plant seeds for reforming it. "After all," Adam Grant opined in *Think Again,* "the purpose of learning isn't to affirm our beliefs; it's to evolve our beliefs."[15]

As mentioned earlier, ambivalence can be a prerequisite for a change in thinking patterns. Until you begin to have some doubts about a currently held belief or attitude, it is unlikely to change. Accommodation is an example of the larger principle of *transcend and include.*[16] Prior beliefs are not necessarily rejected and discarded. Instead, that which is positive and useful is integrated into a new way of understanding. Similarly, seemingly opposite truths may be maintained within a higher-order re-solution. A belief that individual people are separate and independent from each other can morph into an understanding of our interconnection and interdependence, much as a grove of seemingly separate aspen trees is actually one enormous organism linked by a complex underground root system.[17] This does not diminish the beauty and uniqueness of the individual trees; it is simply a larger understanding.

It is possible to hold contradictory experiences simultaneously without needing to choose between or resolve them. It is a switch from "yes, but . . . " to "yes, and . . . " thinking. I experience this now as father of a beloved adult child whose journey at the moment seems to have gone terribly awry. I feel hope that he will turn his life around, and simultaneously I experience dread and despair with his present reality. I don't need to place a bet on one side or the other, nor alternate between them. I hold them together in tension, embracing them both as a whole reality.

The same can be true of two seemingly incompatible beliefs that may be embraced together in dialectic tension:

- *Thesis:* Human beings are inherently loving and pro-social by nature.[18]
- *Antithesis:* Human beings are inherently selfish and antisocial by nature.[19]

Neither proposition can be proven conclusively, and both seem to contain some element of truth. Embracing either view over the other can become a self-fulfilling prophecy, inspiring either generous or suspicious behavior toward others that confirms the belief.[20] Can both be true or reconciled?

- *Synthesis:* People have both potentials and continually choose between them.

This "yes, and . . . " synthesis is a third view that holds both propositions to be true, inspiring still different behavior—perhaps to encourage "the better angels of our nature" in oneself and others.

Finally, ambivalence need not be distressing. Individuals and cultures vary in their comfort or discomfort with inconsistency. Distress and psychological symptoms are linked not so much to the objective presence of ambivalence, but to acceptance of it and ability to manage conflicting motivations. The contemplative practice of mindfulness serves to "clean the lens" and transcend dualistic, judgmental thinking.[21] There is also less need to resolve or stress about ambivalence when you have meaning and creativity in other areas of your life. Perhaps this is why ambivalence often becomes more of a familiar friend as we age.

SOME PERSONAL REFLECTIONS

In researching and working on this book over many months, I realized, as I said in the Preface, that it is actually a topic I have been studying throughout my career. Ambivalence lies at the heart of addiction, a fascinating phenomenon that I have been researching and treating since I was introduced to the field in 1973. Behavioral self-control is all about steering a course through conflicting motivations.[22] Getting unstuck from ambivalence has been a central issue in our counseling method of motivational interviewing.[23]

I have also become much more aware of the role that ambivalence has played at key junctures throughout my life. Here are just a few examples.[24] The untimely death of my young sister when I was 13 shook the foundations of my childhood faith. Who is this God who allows or perhaps even causes such things to happen? A synthesis began for me with our pastor who attempted no explanation, but whose silent tight embrace conveyed that God is intimately present with us in our suffering.[25] I entered college intending to pursue pastoral ministry, but found myself drawn to and majoring in psychology instead. I was also vacillating between music and psychology as possible careers, a candy store choice between passions. My home base in vocational aptitude is *artistic,* so music would have been a natural choice for me, but I chose psychology instead as my career path. The next-door neighbor to artistic on a career interest circumplex is *investigative*—inquiring, analyzing, researching—and that's how my scientific work unfolded, with a dash of creativity in writing and exploring new ideas. Nevertheless music has continued to enrich my life and in retirement I have had time to try my hand at choral composition. Deciding whether to marry was an ambivalent journey to a lifelong soulmate. Chapter 6 described my unconscious struggle with whether we would have children. After being tenured as a psychology professor (thesis), a vivid experience prompted me to wonder whether I had taken the wrong road and should resign my faculty position to go to seminary (antithesis). A series of searching conversations with respected mentors and pastors led to a synthesis that my work was already an important form of ministry, so I found myself in the doorway between psychology and religion passing things back and forth.[26] A different choice at any of these and other passages would have profoundly altered the course of my life.

Ambivalence is not always best resolved. A longstanding tension for me is keeping work in balance with relationships and other life values. I enjoy my work enough that it can expand to fill every available space of time. I first had to learn *don't say yes when you want to say no*.[27] The opportunities continued to expand sufficiently that the challenge for me became *don't say yes when you want to say yes*. Once when I was complaining to a friend about my self-imposed volume and stress of work she suggested, "Perhaps you can just learn to enjoy running on the edge." It's an image that helped: staying not too close to the cliff edge while enjoying the view. I am grateful for the work of a psychologist. Few are as privileged in the course of a lifetime to get to know so many people at an intimate personal level. Yet when I retired I turned in my license to practice, and let go of personal involvement in research. Now I enjoy being an unemployed writer.

LOOKING BACK: AMBIVALENCE IN PERSPECTIVE

In this book, I have tried to pull together for you what I have learned along the way as well as some insights from intriguing research contributed by others. The word *ambivalence* itself is only a century old. It differs from not caring (indifference) and not knowing (ignorance or ambiguity); indeed it emerges only when you do know, care, and have competing motives. It is the experience of simultaneously looking in different directions, like the Roman god Janus, and valuing the alternatives.

There are various "flavors" of ambivalence and particular words by which you can talk yourself into or out of change. There are various levels at which conflict can emerge, generating ambivalence: your immediate thoughts, feelings, and actions; your beliefs, attitudes, and core values. There are some traps to beware when you navigate ambivalence, including:

- Temptation to leave the journey prematurely, taking an early exit of univalence
- Negativity bias that assigns greater importance to fears
- Unconscious motives that can tip the balance
- Preferring immediate or short-term results
- Choosing based on identification
- Binary thinking that sees only two possibilities
- Selective attention to evidence in only one direction

There are also strong social pressures of conformity, authority, and persuasion. Psychological reactance is a built-in human tendency, when given advice, to disregard it or do the opposite, even when you agree with it. Such social influences can operate below your awareness, conveyed in tone of voice or subtleties of language. Unconscious motives and implicit biases can also create ambivalence and bias its resolution.

Objective ambivalence—the mere presence of simultaneous pros and cons—is common and not inherently distressing. In fact, ambivalence is a normal step toward a change in belief or behavior. How upsetting ambivalence will be for you depends on other factors, including time pressure and some personality traits such as openness to experience and need for consistency or closure.

Responses to ambivalence or regret tend to fall into two broad classes: shutting down (inaction, avoidance) and taking action. Being clear on your most important values can help you in resolving ambivalence, as can getting the big picture by simultaneously considering the pros and cons. Once you have settled on a clear direction, a key is to keep moving on that path, rather than being derailed by ambivalence.

Not an unusual event, ambivalence is an ordinary daily experience when choosing among alternatives. Human feelings are richly mixed, as are the motives that impel you on your way. In this sense, ambivalence is the crucible in which you compound your present and future. The experience is so familiar that it can be taken for granted. The inner committee deliberates, sometimes in the foreground but more often in the back rooms of consciousness, with a rich vocabulary to express and resolve seeming contradictions. The topics of discussion range from simple choices—do this or that, believe this or that—to conflicts that reach to your very depths, challenging and shaping who you are. It is exemplified by Tevye in *Fiddler on the Roof,* wrestling with change: "On the one hand . . . and on the other hand." In relationships and public discourse, ambivalence is the dance of persuasion and negotiation by which decisions are reached together.

For both individuals and groups, it is the more contentious topics that tend to capture attention. Yet the ongoing process of evaluating and choosing is the everyday workplace of ambivalence. There is skill involved in continuing to explore the terrain of simultaneous pros and cons long enough to find your way through it.

In the end, ambivalence can be embraced as a gift, a privilege of choosing among possible selves and futures. The experience of ambivalence can awaken you to milestones by which your values are both expressed and shaped, perhaps making some of the most consequential decisions of your life. It is the rich experience of being human: contemplating different possible paths and consciously choosing which you will take. From that perspective, ambivalence is the very essence of being human.

Notes

CHAPTER 1. I WANT IT AND I DON'T

1. S. A. Shapiro. (1968). "The Ambivalent Animal: Man in the Contemporary British and American Novel." *Centennial Review, 12*(1), 1–22.
2. Y. M. Baek. (2010). "An Integrative Model of Ambivalence." *Social Science Journal, 47*(3), 609–629.
3. C. Sedikides, T. Wildschut, J. Arndt, & C. Routledge. (2008). "Nostalgia: Past, Present and Future." *Current Directions in Psychological Science, 17*(5), 304–307.
4. C. Routledge, J. Arndt, T. Wildschut, C. Sedikides, C. M. Hart, J. Juhl, A. J. J. M. Vingerhoets, & W. Schlotz. (2011). "The Past Makes the Present Meaningful: Nostalgia as an Existential Resource." *Journal of Personality and Social Psychology, 101*(3), 638–652.
5. Recorded by Billy Ray Cyrus. An earlier country-western song recorded by Billy Walker had the tag line "I'm So Miserable without You It's Like Having You Around."
6. H. Segal. (2019). "The Achievement of Ambivalence." *Common Knowledge, 25*(1–3), 51–62.
7. F. S. Fitzgerald. (1936, February). "The Crack-Up." *Esquire,* p. 41.
8. T. J. Rudolph & E. Popp. (2007). "An Information Processing Theory of Ambivalence." *Political Psychology, 28*(5), 563–585.

9. C. T. Fong. (2006). "The Effects of Emotional Ambivalence on Creativity." *Academy of Management Journal, 49*(5), 1016–1030.

10. L. Rees, N. B. Rothman, R. Lehavy, & J. Sanchez-Burks. (2013). "The Ambivalent Mind Can Be a Wise Mind: Emotional Ambivalence Increases Judgment Accuracy." *Journal of Experimental Social Psychology, 49*(3), 360–367.

11. Z. D. Peterson & E. Janssen. (2007). "Ambivalent Affect and Sexual Response: The Impact of Co-occurring Positive and Negative Emotions on Subjective and Physiological Sexual Responses to Erotic Stimuli." *Archives of Sexual Behavior, 36*(6), 793–807.

12. D. Engle & H. Arkowitz. (2006). *Ambivalence in Psychotherapy: Facilitating Readiness to Change.* New York: Guilford Press.

13. K. Jonas, P. Broemer, & M. Diehl. (2000). "Attitudinal Ambivalence." *European Review of Social Psychology, 11*(1), 35–74.

14. M. Conner & P. Sparks. (2002). "Ambivalence and Attitudes." *European Review of Social Psychology, 12*(1), 37–70.

CHAPTER 2. FOUR FLAVORS OF AMBIVALENCE

1. J. T. Larsen & A. P. McGraw. (2014). "The Case for Mixed Emotions." *Social and Personality Psychology Compass, 8*(6), 263–274.

2. S. M. Ersner-Hershfield, J. A. Mikels, S. J. Sullivan, & L. L. Carstensen. (2008). "Poignancy: Mixed Emotional Experience in the Face of Meaningful Endings." *Journal of Personality and Social Psychology, 94*(1), 158–167.

3. J. Tierney & R. F. Baumeister. (2021). *The Power of Bad: How the Negativity Effect Rules Us and How We Can Rule It.* New York: Penguin Books.

4. William Blake, "Auguries of Innocence."

5. M. Conner & C. J. Armitage. (2008). "Attitudinal Ambivalence." In W. D. Crano & R. Prislin (Eds.), *Frontiers of Social Psychology: Attitudes and Attitude Change* (pp. 261–286). New York: Psychology Press.

6. The song lyric is from Dan Hicks, "How Can I Miss You When You Won't Go Away?"

7. You may be curious about the outcome for this couple. There is something about an ambivalence story that draws us in, and you want to know what happens. The purpose of this case illustration is to provide an example of a common Go-No ambivalence. Suffice it to say that they remained in therapy for more than a year and did stay together, with significant reduction in broken glassware.

CHAPTER 3. THE LANGUAGE OF AMBIVALENCE

1. P. Ekman & W. V. Friesen. (1969). "Nonverbal Leakage and Clues to Deception." *Psychiatry Journal for the Study of Interpersonal Processes, 32*(1), 88–106.

    M. J. Heisel & M. Mongrain. (2004). "Facial Expressions and Ambivalence: Looking for Conflict in All the Right Faces." *Journal of Nonverbal Behavior, 28*(1), 35–52.

2. I. K. Schneider, A. Eerland, F. van Harreveld, M. Rotteveel, J. van der Pligt, N. van der Stoep, & R. A. Zwaan. (2013). "One Way and the Other: The Bidirectional Relationship between Ambivalence and Body Movement." *Psychological Science, 24*(3), 319–325.

3. C. C. DiClemente, D. Schlundt, & L. Gemmell. (2004). "Readiness and Stages of Change in Addiction Treatment." *American Journal on Addictions, 13,* 103–119.

    J. O. Prochaska, J. Norcross, & C. DiClemente. (1994). *Changing for Good: A Revolutionary Six-Stage Program for Overcoming Bad Habits and Moving Your Life Positively Forward.* New York: Avon Books.

4. C. J. Armitage, R. Povey, & M. A. Arden. (2003). "Evidence for Discontinuity Patterns across the Stages of Change: A Role for Attitudinal Ambivalence." *Psychology and Health, 18*(3), 373–386.

5. R. F. Baumeister, T. F. Heatherton, & D. M. Tice. (1994). *Losing Control: How and Why People Fail at Self-Regulation.* New York: Academic Press.

6. P. C. Amrhein. (2004). "How Does Motivational Interviewing Work? What Client Talk Reveals." *Journal of Cognitive Psychotherapy, 18*(4), 323–336.

W. R. Miller & S. Rollnick. (2013). *Motivational Interviewing: Helping People Change* (3rd ed.). New York: Guilford Press.

7. Our research on self-motivational statements began with W. R. Miller. (1983). "Motivational Interviewing with Problem Drinkers." *Behavioural Psychotherapy, 11,* 147–172.

8. D. J. Bem. (1972). "Self-Perception Theory." In L. Berkowitz (Ed.), *Advances in Experimental Social Psychology* (Vol. 6, pp. 1–62). New York: Academic Press.

9. M. Magill, M. H. Bernstein, A. Hoadley, B. Borsari, T. R. Apodaca, J. Gaume, & J. S. Tonigan. (2019). "Do What You Say and Say What You Are Going to Do: A Preliminary Meta-Analysis of Client Change and Sustain Talk Subtypes in Motivational Interviewing." *Psychotherapy Research, 29*(7), 860–869.

10. C. Khambatta & R. Barbaro. (2020). *Mastering Diabetes: The Revolutionary Method to Reverse Insulin Resistance Permanently.* New York: Penguin Random House.

CHAPTER 4. SOURCES OF AMBIVALENCE

1. M. Rokeach. (1973). *The Nature of Human Values.* New York: Free Press.

2. Ibid, p. 237.

3. Ibid, p. 238.

4. L. A. Penner. (1971). "Interpersonal Attraction toward a Black Person as a Function of Value Importance." *Personality: An International Journal, 2*(2), 175–187.

5. Rokeach called these "terminal" values, the end states we pursue.

6. D. Brooks. (2015). *The Road to Character.* New York: Random House.

7. Thomas Merton further recognized a "True Self" distinct from the attitudes, beliefs, and values that we tend to identify as "me." T. Merton. (1961). *New Seeds of Contemplation.* New York: New Directions.

8. This paraphrased story was originally told by David Premack (1972) in his article, "Mechanisms of Self-Control" in W. A. Hunt (Ed.), *Learning Mechanisms in Smoking* (pp. 107–123). Chicago: Aldine.

9. D. A. Snow & R. Machalek. (1984). "The Sociology of Conversion." *Annual Review of Sociology, 10,* 167–190.

A. Buckser & S. D. Glazier (Eds.). (2003). *The Anthropology of Religious Conversion.* Lanham, MD: Rowman & Littlefield.

10. M. G. Pratt. (1988). "To Be or Not to Be: Central Questions in Organizational Identification." In D. Whetten & P. Godfrey (Eds.), *Identity in Organizations: Developing Theory through Conversations* (pp. 171–207). Thousand Oaks, CA: Sage.

11. M. Pratt. (2000). "The Good, the Bad, and the Ambivalent: Managing Identification among Amway Distributors." *Administrative Science Quarterly, 45,* 456–493.

12. J. W. Fowler. (1993). "Alcoholics Anonymous and Faith Development." In B. S. McCrady & W. R. Miller (Eds.), *Research on Alcoholics Anonymous: Opportunities and Alternatives* (pp. 113–135). New Brunswick, NJ: Rutgers Center of Alcohol Studies.

13. St. Teresa of Avila. (2003). *The Interior Castle* (M. Starr, Trans.). New York: Riverhead Books, pp. 157–158.

14. J. Tierney & R. F. Baumeister. (2021). *The Power of Bad: How the Negativity Effect Rules Us and How We Can Rule It.* New York: Penguin Books.

15. J. T. Cacioppo, W. L. Gardner, & G. G. Berntson. (1997). "Beyond Bipolar Conceptualizations and Measures: The Case of Attitudes and Evaluative Space." *Personality and Social Psychology Review, 1*(1), 3–25.

16. J. R. Priester & R. E. Petty. (1996). "The Gradual Threshold Model of Ambivalence: Relating the Positive and Negative Bases of Attitudes to Subjective Ambivalence." *Journal of Personality and Social Psychology, 71*(3), 431–449.

17. M. Magill, T. R. Apodaca, B. Borsari, J. Gaume, A. Hoadley, R. E. F. Gordon, . . . T. Moyers. (2018). "A Meta-Analysis of Motivational Interviewing Process: Technical, Relational, and Conditional Process Models of Change." *Journal of Consulting and Clinical Psychology, 86*(2), 140–157.

18. S. Cain. (2013). *Quiet: The Power of Introverts in a World That Can't Stop Talking.* New York: Random House.

CHAPTER 5. SOCIAL INFLUENCES

1. An engaging tale of exploring life outside his reference group bubble is told by Kenneth Stern in his book *Republican Like Me: How I Left the Liberal Bubble and Learned to Love the Right* (2017, New York: Harper Collins). The title sounds like a conversion story of flipping political parties, but it is much better than that. Through spending a year outside his comfort zone, Stern discovered how alike people are regardless of political affiliation.

2. S. Asch. (1955). "Opinions and Social Pressure." *Scientific American, 193*(5), 31–35.

    S. E. Asch. (1956). "Studies of Independence and Conformity: I. A Minority of One against a Unanimous Majority." *Psychological Monographs: General and Applied, 70*(9), 1–70.

3. D. Peabody. (1967). "Trait Inferences: Evaluative and Descriptive Aspects." *Journal of Personality and Social Psychology Monographs, 7*(4, Pt. 2, Whole No. 644).

    P. De Boeck. (1978). "On the Evaluative Factor in the Trait Scales of Peabody's Study of Trait Inferences." *Journal of Personality and Social Psychology, 36*(6), 619–621.

4. The story is detailed in L. Festinger, H. W. Riecken, & S. Schachter. (1956). *When Prophecy Fails*. Minneapolis: University of Minnesota Press.

5. M. Conner & P. Sparks. (2002). "Ambivalence and Attitudes." *European Review of Social Psychology, 12*(1), 37–70.

6. Blaise Pascal, *Pensées*.

7. W. R. Miller & S. Rollnick. (2004). "Talking Oneself into Change: Motivational Interviewing, Stages of Change, and Therapeutic Process." *Journal of Cognitive Psychotherapy, 18,* 299–308.

8. S. Milmoe, R. Rosenthal, H. T. Blane, M. E. Chafetz, & I. Wolf. (1967). "The Doctor's Voice: Postdictor of Successful Referral of Alcoholic Patients." *Journal of Abnormal Psychology, 72*(1), 78–84.

9. J. Bernstein, E. Bernstein, K. Tassiopoulos, T. Heeren, S. Levenson, & R. Hingson. (2005). "Brief Motivational Intervention at a Clinic Visit Reduces Cocaine and Heroin Use." *Drug and Alcohol Dependence, 77,* 49–59.

M. E. Chafetz. (1961). "A Procedure for Establishing Therapeutic Contact with the Alcoholic." *Quarterly Journal of Studies on Alcohol, 22,* 325–328.

M. E. Chafetz, H. T. Blane, H. S. Abram, J. H. Golner, E. L. Hastie, & W. Meyers. (1962). "Establishing Treatment Relations with Alcoholics." *Journal of Nervous and Mental Disease, 134,* 395–409.

10. N. Ambady, D. LaPlante, T. Nguyen, R. Rosenthal, N. Chaumeton, & W. Levinson. (2002). "Surgeons' Tone of Voice: A Clue to Malpractice History." *Surgery, 132,* 5–9.

11. S. S. Brehm & J. W. Brehm. (1981). *Psychological Reactance: A Theory of Freedom and Control.* New York: Academic Press.

   S. A. Rains. (2013). "The Nature of Psychological Reactance Revisited: A Meta-Analytic Review." *Human Communication Research, 39*(1), 47–73.

12. A. C. de Almeida Neto. (2017). "Understanding Motivational Interviewing: An Evolutionary Perspective." *Evolutionary Psychological Science, 3*(4), 379–389.

13. M. Polacsek, E. M. Rogers, W. G. Woodall, H. Delaney, D. Wheeler, & N. Rao. (2001). "MADD Victim Impact Panels and Stages-of-Change in Drunk-Driving Prevention." *Journal of Studies on Alcohol, 62*(3), 344–350.

14. W. G. Woodall, H. Delaney, E. Rogers, & D. Wheeler. (2000). "A Randomized Trial of Victim Impact Panels' DWI Deterrence Effectiveness." *Alcoholism: Clinical & Experimental Research, 24 (Supplement),* 113A (Abstract 637).

CHAPTER 6. OUT OF THE DEPTHS

1. I originally told this story in W. R. Miller & J. C'de Baca(2001), *Quantum Change: When Epiphanies and Sudden Insights Transform Ordinary Lives* (New York: Guilford Press). Copyright © 2001 The Guilford Press. Used by permission.

2. Malcolm Gladwell. (2007). *Blink: The Power of Thinking without Thinking.* New York: Little, Brown, p. 155.

3. J. A. Bargh & T. L. Chartrand. (1999). "The Unbearable Automaticity of Being." *American Psychologist, 54*, 462–479.

4. L. Quillian. (2008). "Does Unconscious Racism Exist?" *Social Psychology Quarterly, 71*(1), 6–11.

5. N. L. Quenk. (2002). *Was That Really Me? How Everyday Stress Brings Out Our Hidden Personality*. Mountain View, CA: Davies-Black.

6. Y. M. Baek. (2010). "An Integrative Model of Ambivalence." *Social Science Journal, 47*(3), 609–629.

7. P. Ekman & W. V. Friesen. (1969). "Nonverbal Leakage and Clues to Deception." *Psychiatry Journal for the Study of Interpersonal Processes, 32*(1), 88–106.

8. C. Butler & S. Rollnick. (1996). "Missing the Meaning and Provoking Resistance." *Family Practice, 13*(1), 106–109.

9. Y. M. Baek. (2010). "An Integrative Model of Ambivalence." *Social Science Journal, 47*(3), 609–629.

10. A. Christensen, K. A. Eldridge, A. B. Catta-Preta, V. R. Lim, & R. Santagata. (2006). "Cross-Cultural Consistence of the Demand/Withdraw Interaction Pattern in Couples." *Journal of Marriage and Family, 68*(4), 1029–1044.

11. I described Julia's case in more detail in W. R. Miller & S. Rollnick. (2013). *Motivational Interviewing: Helping People Change* (3rd ed.). New York: Guilford Press.

CHAPTER 7. CONSEQUENCES OF AMBIVALENCE

1. J. E. Holoubek & A. B. Holoubek. (1996). "Blood, Sweat and Fear. 'A Classification of Hematidrosis'." *Journal of Medicine, 27*(3–4), 115–133.

2. F. van Harreveld, H. U. Nohlen, & I. K. Schneider. (2015). "The ABC of Ambivalence: Affective, Behavioral, and Cognitive Consequences of Attitudinal Conflict." *Advances in Experimental Social Psychology, 52*, 285–324.

3. Ibid.

4. S. Schachter & J. Singer. (1962). "Cognitive, Social and Physiological

Determinants of Emotional State." *Psychological Review, 69*(5), 379–399.

5. R. E. Kelly, W. Mansell, & A. M. Wood. (2015). "Goal Conflict and Well-Being: A Review and Hierarchical Model of Goal Conflict, Ambivalence, Self-Discrepancy and Self-Concordance." *Personality and Individual Differences, 85,* 212–229.

6. K. Jonas, P. Broemer, & M. Diehl. (2000). "Attitudinal Ambivalence." *European Review of Social Psychology, 11*(1), 35–74.

7. K. Jonas, M. Diehl, & P. Broemer. (1997). "Effects of Attitudinal Ambivalence on Information Processing and Attitude-Intention Consistency." *Journal of Experimental Social Psychology, 33,* 190–210.

8. C. J. Armitage & M. Conner. (2000). "Social Cognition Models and Health Behaviour: A Structured Review." *Psychology & Health, 15*(2), 173–189.

9. M. Conner & P. Sparks. (2002). "Ambivalence and Attitudes." *European Review of Social Psychology, 12*(1), 37–70.

M. Conner, R. Povey, P. Sparks, R. James, & R. Shepherd. (2003). "Moderating Role of Attitudinal Ambivalence within the Theory of Planned Behaviour." *Journal of Analytical Psychology, 42*(1), 75–94.

10. I. K. Schneider, M. Gillebaart, & A. Mattes. (2019). "Meta-Analytic Evidence for Ambivalence Resolution as a Key Process in Effortless Self-Control." *Journal of Experimental Social Psychology, 85*(November), 103846.

S. Rollnick, W. R. Miller, & C. C. Butler. (2021). *Motivational Interviewing in Health Care: Helping Patients Change Behavior* (2nd ed.). New York: Guilford Press. [Manuscript submitted for publication.]

11. M. J. Apter. (1982). *The Experience of Motivation: The Theory of Psychological Reversals.* New York: Academic Press.

12. J. Cassidy & L. J. Berlin. (1994). "The Insecure/Ambivalent Pattern of Attachment: Theory and Research." *Child Development, 65*(4), 971–991.

13. Alcoholics Anonymous World Services. (2001). *Alcoholics Anonymous: The Story of How Many Thousands of Men and Women Have Recovered from Alcoholism* (4th ed.). New York: Author.

R. Rohr. (2011). *Breathing under Water: Spirituality and the Twelve Steps.* Cincinnati, OH: St. Anthony Messenger Press.

14. T. Merton. (1953). *The Sign of Jonas*. Orlando, FL: Harcourt.

15. F. van Harreveld, H. U. Nohlen, & I. K. Schneider. (2015). "The ABC of Ambivalence: Affective, Behavioral, and Cognitive Consequences of Attitudinal Conflict." *Advances in Experimental Social Psychology, 52,* 285–324.

16. C. T. Fong. (2006). "The Effects of Emotional Ambivalence on Creativity." *Academy of Management Journal, 5,* 1016–1030.

17. R. G. Tedeschi & L. G. Calhoun. (2004). "Posttraumatic Growth: Conceptual Foundations and Empirical Evidence." *Psychological Inquiry, 15*(1), 1–18.

L. G. Calhoun & R. G. Tedeschi (Eds.). (2014). *Handbook of Posttraumatic Growth: Research and Practice*. New York: Psychology Press.

18. N. B. Rothman, M. G. Pratt, L. Rees, & T. J. Vogus. (2017). "Understanding the Dual Nature of Ambivalence: Why and When Ambivalence Leads to Good and Bad Outcomes." *Academy of Management Annals, 11*(1), 33–72.

19. M. M. Tugade, B. L. Fredrickson, & L. F. Barrett. (2004). "Psychological Resilience and Positive Emotional Granularity: Examining the Benefits of Positive Emotions on Coping and Health." *Journal of Personality, 72*(6), 1161–1190.

20. Loving detachment is a familiar component of 12-step programs for family members of people suffering from addictions. Participation in groups such as Al-Anon has been found to help affected family members reduce negative emotions and physical symptoms. W. R. Miller, R. J. Meyers, & J. S. Tonigan. (1999). "Engaging the Unmotivated in Treatment for Alcohol Problems: A Comparison of Three Strategies for Intervention through Family Members." *Journal of Consulting and Clinical Psychology, 67,* 688–697.

CHAPTER 8. INDIVIDUAL DIFFERENCES

1. L. R. Goldberg. (1993). "The Structure of Phenotypic Personality Traits." *American Psychologist, 48*(1), 26–34.

2. A common measure of this preference is the Judging-Perceiving scale of the Myers-Briggs Type Indicator. I. B. Myers & P. B. Myers. (1995). *Gifts Differing: Understanding Personality Type.* Mountain View, CA: Davies-Black.

3. N. D. Volkow, G. F. Koob, & T. McLellan. (2016). "Neurobiologic Advances from the Brain Disease Model of Addiction." *New England Journal of Medicine, 374,* 363–371.

4. W. Mischel, Y. Shoda, & M. I. Rodriguez. (1989). "Delay of Gratification in Children." *Science, 244*(4907), 933–938.

5. W. Mischel, Y. Shoda, & P. K. Peake. (1988). "The Nature of Adolescent Competencies Predicted by Preschool Delay of Gratification." *Journal of Personality and Social Psychology, 54*(4), 687–696.

Y. Shoda, W. Mischel, & P. K. Peake. (1990). "Predicting Adolescent Cognitive and Self-Regulatory Competencies from Preschool Delay of Gratification: Identifying Diagnostic Conditions." *Developmental Psychology, 26*(6), 978–986.

6. T. R. Schlam, N. L. Wilson, Y. Shoda, W. Mischel, & O. Ayduk. (2013). "Preschoolers' Delay of Gratification Predicts Their Body Mass 30 Years Later." *Journal of Pediatrics, 162*(1), 90–93.

7. A. L. Odum, R. J. Becker, J. M. Haynes, A. Galizio, C. C. J. Frye, H. Downey, ... D. M. Perez. (2020). "Delay Discounting of Different Outcomes: Review and Theory." *Journal of the Experimental Analysis of Behavior, 113*(3), 657–679.

8. W. K. Bickel & L. A. Marsch. (2001). "Toward a Behavioral Economic Understanding of Drug Dependence: Delay Discounting Processes." *Addiction, 96*(1), 73–86.

9. C. G. Jung. (1921/1971). *Psychological Types* (G. Adler & R. F. C. Hully, Trans.). Princeton, NJ: Princeton University Press.

10. I. R. Newby-Clark, I. McGregor, & M. P. Zanna. (2002). "Thinking and Caring about Cognitive Inconsistency: When and for Whom Does Attitudinal Ambivalence Feel Uncomfortable?" *Journal of Personality and Social Psychology, 82*(2), 157–166.

11. R. B. Cialdini, M. R. Trost, & T. J. Newsom. (1995). "Preference for Consistency: The Development of a Valid Measure and the Discovery of Surprising Behavioral Implications." *Journal of Personality and Social Psychology, 69*(2), 318–328.

12. Ibid.

CHAPTER 9. RESPONDING TO AMBIVALENCE

1. T. S. Kuhn. (1962). *The Structure of Scientific Revolutions*. Chicago: University of Chicago Press.

2. M. Planck. (2012). *The Origin and Development of the Quantum Theory: With "A Scientific Autobiography."* Hardpress Publishing.

3. Shakespeare's *Hamlet*, Act 3, Scene 1.

4. F. van Harreveld, H. U. Nohlen, & I. K. Schneider. (2015). "The ABC of Ambivalence: Affective, Behavioral, and Cognitive Consequences of Attitudinal Conflict." *Advances in Experimental Social Psychology, 52*, 285–324. Quotation from page 304.

5. J. E. Loder. (1981). *The Transforming Moment: Understanding Convictional Experiences*. New York: Harper & Row.

  J. W. Fowler. (1981). *Stages of Faith: The Psychology of Development and the Quest for Meaning*. San Francisco: Harper & Row.

6. J. W. Fowler. (1993). "Alcoholics Anonymous and Faith Development." In B. S. McCrady & W. R. Miller (Eds.), *Research on Alcoholics Anonymous: Opportunities and Alternatives* (pp. 113–135). New Brunswick, NJ: Rutgers Center of Alcohol Studies. Quotation from page 132.

  A. Forcehimes. (2004). "De Profundis: Spiritual Transformations in Alcoholics Anonymous." *Journal of Clinical Psychology, 60*, 503–517.

7. M. E. Pagano, W. L. White, J. F. Kelly, R. L. Stout, & J. S. Tonigan. (2013). "The 10-Year Course of Alcoholics Anonymous Participation and Long-Term Outcomes: A Follow-Up Study of Outpatient Subjects in Project MATCH." *Substance Abuse, 34*(1), 51–59.

8. W. R. Miller. (2004). "The Phenomenon of Quantum Change." *Journal of Clinical Psychology, 60*(5), 453–460.

  W. R. Miller & J. C'de Baca. (2001). *Quantum Change: When Epiphanies and Sudden Insights Transform Ordinary Lives*. New York: Guilford Press.

9. I. Katz, D. C. Glass, D. J. Lucido, & J. Farber. (1977). "Ambivalence, Guilt, and the Denigration of a Physically Handicapped Victim." *Journal of Personality, 45*(3), 419–429.

10. J. Nowinski. (2004). "Evil by Default: The Origins of Dark Visions." *Journal of Clinical Psychology/In Session, 60*, 519–530.

11. D. Searls. (2017). *The Inkblots: Hermann Rorschach, His Iconic Test, and the Power of Seeing.* New York: Crown.

12. L. Festinger, H. W. Riecken, & S. Schachter. (1956). *When Prophecy Fails.* Minneapolis: University of Minnesota Press.

13. K. M. Douglas, R. M. Sutton, & A. Cichocka. (2017). "The Psychology of Conspiracy Theories." *Current Directions in Psychological Science, 26*(6), 538–542.

14. S. L. Bem. (1981). "Gender Schema Theory: A Cognitive Account of Sex Typing." *Psychological Review, 88,* 354–364.

15. W. R. Miller & J. C'de Baca. (2001). *Quantum Change: When Epiphanies and Sudden Insights Transform Ordinary Lives.* New York: Guilford Press.

16. W. R. Miller, R. G. Sovereign, & B. Krege. (1988). "Motivational Interviewing with Problem Drinkers: II. The Drinker's Check-Up as a Preventive Intervention." *Behavioural Psychotherapy, 16,* 251–268.

    W. R. Miller, A. Zweben, C. C. DiClemente, & R. G. Rychtarik. (1992). *Motivational Enhancement Therapy Manual: A Clinical Research Guide for Therapists Treating Individuals with Alcohol Abuse and Dependence* (Vol. 2, Project MATCH Monograph Series). Rockville, MD: National Institute on Alcohol Abuse and Alcoholism.

17. K. Wilber. (2007). *The Integral Vision.* Boston: Shambhala.

    K. Wilber. (2017). *The Religion of Tomorrow: A Vision for the Future of the Great Traditions—More Inclusive, More Comprehensive, More Complete.* Boulder, CO: Shambhala.

18. A. Grant. (2021). *Think Again: The Power of Knowing What You Don't Know.* New York: Viking.

CHAPTER 10. GETTING CLEAR ON YOUR VALUES

1. H. Markus & P. Nurius. (1986). "Possible Selves." *American Psychologist, 41*(9), 954–969.

2. C. R. Rogers. (1951). *Client-Centered Therapy.* New York: Houghton-Mifflin.

3. C. R. Rogers. (1959). "A Theory of Therapy, Personality, and Interpersonal Relationships as Developed in the Client-Centered Framework." In S. Koch (Ed.), *Psychology: The Study of a Science. Vol. 3.*

Formulations of the Person and the Social Contexts (pp. 184–256). New York: McGraw-Hill.

4. James Thurber's short story, "The Secret Life of Walter Mitty," is a classic example of dream selves. So also is Snoopy's imaginary persona as the Flying Ace fighter pilot in the *Charlie Brown* cartoon series by Charles Schultz.

5. M. Pratt. (2000). "The Good, the Bad, and the Ambivalent: Managing Identification among Amway Distributors." *Administrative Science Quarterly, 45,* 456–493.

6. "Carrot and stick" is sometimes mistakenly taken to mean reward (carrot) or punishment (stick). In fact, the image is of an enticing treat dangling on a string at the end of a stick, keeping it out in front of but just beyond the reach of a donkey in order to keep it moving forward.

7. J. Nowinski. (2004). "Evil by Default: The Origins of Dark Visions." *Journal of Clinical Psychology/In Session, 60,* 519–530.

   A. Haley & Malcolm X. (1964). *The Autobiography of Malcolm X.* New York: Ballantine.

8. C. G. Jung. (1959). *Aion: Researches into the Phenomenology of the Self* (*Collected works of C. G. Jung*, Vol. 9, Part ii). Princeton, NJ: Princeton University Press.

9. N. L. Quenk. (2002). *Was That Really Me? How Everyday Stress Brings Out Our Hidden Personality.* Mountain View, CA: Davies-Black.

10. Y. M. Baek. (2010). An Integrative Model of Ambivalence. *Social Science Journal, 47*(3), 609–629.

11. Shakespeare's *Hamlet,* Act I, Scene 3.

12. C. R. Rogers. (1961). *On Becoming a Person: A Therapist's View of Psychotherapy.* Boston: Houghton Mifflin.

13. K. M. Sheldon & T. Kasser. (2001). "Goals, Congruence and Positive Well-Being: New Empirical Support for Humanistic Theories." *Journal of Humanistic Psychology, 41*(1), 30–50.

14. R. E. Kelly, W. Mansell, & A. M. Wood. (2015). "Goal Conflict and Well-Being: A Review and Hierarchical Model of Goal Conflict, Ambivalence, Self-Discrepancy and Self-Concordance." *Personality and Individual Differences, 85,* 212–229.

15. W. R. Miller, J. C'de Baca, D. B. Matthews, & P. L. Wilbourne.

(2001). *Personal Values Card Sort*. Department of Psychology, University of New Mexico. Albuquerque, NM.

16. W. R. Miller, J. C'de Baca, D. B. Matthews, & P. L. Wilbourne. (2001). "Personal Values Card Sort." Retrieved from *https://motivationalinterviewing.org/sites/default/files/valuescardsort_0.pdf*.

17. W. R. Miller & J. C'de Baca. (2001). *Quantum Change: When Epiphanies and Sudden Insights Transform Ordinary Lives*. New York: Guilford Press.

CHAPTER 11. GETTING THE BIG PICTURE

1. Peter Abelard's 12th century *Sic et Non* (*Yes and No*) is a classic example, weighing the merits of conflicting arguments on theological questions.

2. B. Franklin. (1904). "Moral or Prudential Algebra: Letter to Joseph Priestly (September 19, 1772)." In J. Bigelow (Ed.), *The Works of Benjamin Franklin, Vol. V Letters and Misc. Writings 1768–1772* (Vol. 5). New York: Putnam. In the original, Franklin capitalized all nouns as was a custom of the time. I removed this convention as it is unfamiliar to modern readers.

3. I. L. Janis & L. Mann. (1977). *Decision Making: A Psychological Analysis of Conflict, Choice and Commitment*. New York: Free Press. Irving Janis taught psychology at Yale University for 40 years, and is better known for his research on *groupthink*—how group conformity restricts creativity and biases individual judgment.

4. I. L. Janis. (1989). *Crucial Decisions: Leadership in Policymaking and Crisis Management*. New York: Free Press.

5. W. R. Miller. (1983). "Motivational Interviewing with Problem Drinkers." *Behavioural Psychotherapy, 11*, 147–172.

6. W. R. Miller, R. G. Benefield, & J. S. Tonigan. (1993). "Enhancing Motivation for Change in Problem Drinking: A Controlled Comparison of Two Therapist Styles." *Journal of Consulting and Clinical Psychology, 61*, 455–461.

7. B. W. Lundahl, C. Kunz, C. Brownell, D. Tollefson, & B. L. Burke. (2010). "A Meta-Analysis of Motivational Interviewing: Twenty-Five

Years of Empirical Studies." *Research on Social Work Practice, 20*(2), 137–160.

S. Rubak, A. Sandbaek, T. Lauritzen, & B. Christensen. (2005). "Motivational Interviewing: A Systematic Review and Meta-Analysis." *British Journal of General Practice, 55*(513), 305–312.

8. C. G. Chorus. (2010). "A New Model of Random Regret Minimization." *European Journal of Transport and Infrastructure Research, 10*(2), 181–196.

9. H. Bleichrodt & P. P. Wakker. (2015). "Regret Theory: A Bold Alternative to the Alternatives." *The Economic Journal, 125*(583), 493–532.

10. T. Connolly & M. Zeelenberg. (2002). "Regret in Decision Making." *Current Directions in Psychological Science, 11*(6), 212–216.

11. M. Zeelenberg & R. Pieters. (2007). "A Theory of Regret Regulation 1.0." *Journal of Consumer Psychology, 17*(1), 3–18.

12. H. Zehr. (2015). *Changing Lenses: Restorative Justice for Our Times* (25th anniversary ed.). Harrisonburg, VA: Herald Press.

CHAPTER 12. GETTING OUT OF THE WOODS

1. P. C. Amrhein. (1992). "The Comprehension of Quasi-Performance Verbs in Verbal Commitments: New Evidence for Componential Theories of Lexical Meaning." *Journal of Memory and Language, 31,* 756–784.

2. Ibid.

3. W. R. Miller & S. Rollnick. (2013). *Motivational Interviewing: Helping People Change* (3rd ed.). New York: Guilford Press.

4. P. C. Amrhein, W. R. Miller, C. E. Yahne, M. Palmer, & L. Fulcher. (2003). "Client Commitment Language during Motivational Interviewing Predicts Drug Use Outcomes." *Journal of Consulting and Clinical Psychology, 71,* 862–878.

T. B. Moyers, T. Martin, P. J. Christopher, J. M. Houck, J. S. Tonigan, & P. C. Amrhein. (2007). "Client Language as a Mediator of Motivational Interviewing Efficacy: Where Is the Evidence?" *Alcoholism: Clinical and Experimental Research, 31*(10 Suppl), 40s–47s.

5. T. B. Moyers, T. Martin, J. M. Houck, P. J. Christopher, & J. S. Tonigan. (2009). "From In-Session Behaviors to Drinking Outcomes: A Causal Chain for Motivational Interviewing." *Journal of Consulting and Clinical Psychology, 77*(6), 1113–1124.

6. When I was diagnosed, I was referred for a 90-minute lecture on what I needed to do differently, complete with plastic food servings. I sat there thinking, "There must be a more effective way to do this," and I wound up collaborating with a diabetologist colleague, Dr. Marc P. Steinberg, to write *Motivational Interviewing in Diabetes Care* (Guilford Press, 2015).

7. I thank my colleague, Dr. Theresa Moyers, for this clear example.

8. I first described this method in W. R. Miller. (1983). "Motivational Interviewing with Problem Drinkers." *Behavioural Psychotherapy, 11,* 147–172. There are now many books on the subject, including W. R. Miller & S. Rollnick. (2013). *Motivational Interviewing: Helping People Change* (3rd ed.). New York: Guilford Press.

9. B. W. Lundahl, C. Kunz, C. Brownell, D. Tollefson, & B. L. Burke. (2010). "A Meta-Analysis of Motivational Interviewing: Twenty-Five Years of Empirical Studies." *Research on Social Work Practice, 20*(2), 137–160.

S. Rubak, A. Sandbaek, T. Lauritzen, & B. Christensen. (2005). "Motivational Interviewing: A Systematic Review and Meta-Analysis." *British Journal of General Practice, 55*(513), 305–312.

10. J. Strang & J. Mccambridge. (2004). "Can the Practitioner Correctly Predict Outcome in Motivational Interviewing?" *Journal of Substance Abuse Treatment, 27*(1), 83–88.

T. B. Moyers, T. Martin, J. M. Houck, P. J. Christopher, & J. S. Tonigan. (2009). "From In-Session Behaviors to Drinking Outcomes: A Causal Chain for Motivational Interviewing." *Journal of Consulting and Clinical Psychology, 77*(6), 1113–1124.

11. It may be easier to do this with a skillful interviewer, but most of the time people do it on their own. A book designed to help you interview yourself in this way is A. Zuckoff, with B. Gorscak. (2015). *Finding Your Way to Change: How the Power of Motivational Interviewing Can Reveal What You Want and Help You Get There*. New York: Guilford Press.

12. W. R. Miller. (1985). *Living As If: How Positive Faith Can Change Your Life*. Eugene, OR: Wipf & Stock.

W. R. Miller. (2008). *Living As If: Your Road, Your Life*. Carson City, NV: The Change Companies.

CHAPTER 13. EMBRACING AMBIVALENCE

1. S. A. Shapiro. (1968). "The Ambivalent Animal: Man in the Contemporary British and American Novel." *Centennial Review, 12*(1), 1–22.

2. J. O. Prochaska, J. Norcross, & C. DiClemente. (1994). *Changing for Good: A Revolutionary Six-Stage Program for Overcoming Bad Habits and Moving Your Life Positively Forward*. New York: Avon Books.

3. M. G. Pratt & C. K. Barnett. (1997). "Emotions and Unlearning in Amway Recruiting Techniques: Promoting Change through 'Safe' Ambivalence." *Management Learning, 18*(1), 65–88.

4. A. J. Weigert. (1989). "Joyful Disaster: An Ambivalence-Religion Hypothesis." *Sociology of Religion, 50*(1), 73–88.

5. A. J. Weigert. (1991). *Mixed Emotions: Certain Steps toward Understanding Ambivalence*. Albany, NY: State University of New York Press.

6. A. Herman. (2001). *How the Scots Invented the Modern World*. New York: Three Rivers Press.

Presbyterian Church (U.S.A.). (2019–2021). *Book of Order: The Constitution of the Presbyterian Church (U.S.A.)* (Vol. II). Louisville, KY: Office of the General Assembly.

7. N. Plambeck & K. Weber. (2009). "CEO Ambivalence and Responses to Strategic Issues." *Organization Science, 20*(6), 993–1010.

8. S. C. Hayes, V. M. Follette, & M. M. Linehan (Eds.). (2004). *Mindfulness and Acceptance: Expanding the Cognitive-Behavioral Tradition*. New York: Guilford Press.

9. E. L. Worthington Jr. (2003). *Forgiving and Reconciling: Bridges to Wholeness and Hope*. Downers Grove, IL: InterVarsity Press.

10. W. James. (1994/1902). *The Varieties of Religious Experience*. New York: Modern Library Edition.

11. S. Freud. (1928/2010). *The Future of an Illusion*. Seattle, WA: Pacific Publishing Studio.

A. Ellis. (1988). "Is Religiosity Pathological?" *Free Inquiry, 18*, 27–32.

12. R. W. Hood Jr., P. C. Hill, & B. Spilka. (2018). *The Psychology of Religion: An Empirical Approach* (5th ed.). New York: Guilford Press.

13. H. D. Delaney, W. R. Miller, & A. M. Bisonó. (2007). "Religiosity and Spirituality among Psychologists: A Survey of Clinician Members of the American Psychological Association." *Professional Psychology: Research and Practice, 38*(5), 538–546.

14. E. P. Shafranske (Ed.). (1996). *Religion and the Clinical Practice of Psychology*. Washington, DC: American Psychological Association.

W. R. Miller (Ed.). (1999). *Integrating Spirituality into Treatment: Resources for Practitioners*. Washington, DC: American Psychological Association.

15. A. Grant (2021). *Think Again: The Power of Knowing What You Don't Know*. New York: Viking, p. 26.

16. K. Wilber. (2007). *The Integral Vision*. Boston: Shambhala.

17. S. Van Booy. (2013). *The Illusion of Separateness*. New York: HarperCollins.

W. R. Miller & J. C'de Baca. (2001). *Quantum Change: When Epiphanies and Sudden Insights Transform Ordinary Lives*. New York: Guilford Press.

18. W. R. Miller. (2017). *Lovingkindness: Realizing and Practicing Your True Self*. Eugene, OR: Wipf & Stock.

C. R. Rogers. (1962). "The Nature of Man." In S. Doniger (Ed.), *The Nature of Man in Theological and Psychological Perspective* (pp. 91–96). New York: Harper & Brothers.

19. This perspective is vividly conveyed in William Golding's 1954 novel *The Lord of the Flies,* in which children left to their own devices in isolation quickly devolve into brutes.

20. R. A. Jones. (1981). *Self-Fulfilling Prophecies: Social, Psychological, and Physiological Effects of Expectancies*. New York: Psychology Press.

W. R. Miller. (1985). *Living As If: How Positive Faith Can Change Your Life*. Eugene, OR: Wipf & Stock.

21. R. Rohr. (2003). *Everything Belongs: The Gift of Contemplative Prayer.* New York: Crossroads Publishing.

Thich Nhat Hanh. (2015). *The Miracle of Mindfulness: An Introduction to the Practice of Meditation* (Mobi Ho, Trans.). Boston: Beacon Press.

22. R. F. Baumeister, T. F. Heatherton, & D. M. Tice. (1994). *Losing Control: How and Why People Fail at Self-Regulation.* New York: Academic Press.

M. J. Mahoney & C. E. Thoresen. (1974). *Self-Control: Power to the Person.* Monterey, CA: Brooks/Cole.

W. R. Miller & D. J. Atencio. (2008). "Free Will as a Proportion of Variance." In J. Baer, J. C. Kaufman, & R. F. Baumeister (Eds.). *Are We Free? Psychology and Free Will* (pp. 275–295). New York: Oxford University Press.

23. W. R. Miller. (1983). Motivational Interviewing with Problem Drinkers. *Behavioural Psychotherapy, 11,* 147–172.

W. R. Miller & S. Rollnick. (2013). *Motivational Interviewing: Helping People Change* (3rd ed.). New York: Guilford Press.

24. An inside account of some ambivalent turning points is offered in W. R. Miller & L. K. Homer. (2016). *Portals: Two Lives Intertwined by Adoption.* Eugene, OR: Wipf & Stock.

25. R. Rohr. (2011). *Falling Upward: A Spirituality for the Two Halves of Life.* San Francisco: Jossey Bass.

26. W. R. Miller & K. A. Jackson. (2010). *Practical Psychology for Pastors* (2nd ed.). Eugene, OR: Wipf & Stock.

W. R. Miller (Ed.). (1999). *Integrating Spirituality into Treatment: Resources for Practitioners.* Washington, DC: American Psychological Association.

W. R. Miller & H. D. Delaney (Eds.). (2005). *Judeo-Christian Perspectives on Psychology: Human Nature, Motivation and Change.* Washington, DC: American Psychological Association.

27. A 1975 book with this title by Herb Fensterheim and Jean Baer sold millions of copies.

Index

About the Author

William R. Miller, PhD, is Emeritus Distinguished Professor of Psychology and Psychiatry at the University of New Mexico. He has been studying ambivalence for five decades and has personally been living with it for well longer than that. Fundamentally interested in the psychology of change, Dr. Miller is a cofounder of motivational interviewing. The Institute for Scientific Information has listed him as one of the world's most highly cited researchers.